THE ME
IN THE
MIRROR

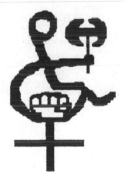

Connie Panzarino

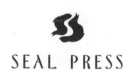

SEAL PRESS

Cover design by Kris Morgan

Book design by Clare Conrad

Cover art, by Connie Panzarino, is a pen and ink blind contour drawing done by hand in 1979. It won several graphic awards in New York shows and galleries and is now owned by Elizabeth Ouwang.

Library of Congress Cataloging-in-Publication Data

Panzarino, Connie, 1947–
  The Me in the Mirror / Connie Panzarino
    p.   cm.
  ISBN 1-878067-45-1 : $12.95
    1. Panzarino, Connie, 1947—Health. 2. Spinal Muscular Atrophy—Patients—United States—Biography. 3. Physically handicapped women—United States—Biography. 4. Lesbians—United States—Biography. I. Title.
  RC935.M95P36   1994   93-41623
  362.1'9674'0092—dc20   CIP
  [B]

Printed in the United States of America
First Printing, May 1994
10 9 8 7 6 5 4 3 2 1

Distributed to the trade by Publishers Group West
Foreign Distribution:
  In Great Britain and Europe: Airlift Book Company, London

*This book is dedicated
to all persons with disabilities
living behind the bars
of the many institutions that still
keep us caged.*

ACKNOWLEDGMENTS

Let me first start with thanking my mother who told me when I was very young that I should write a book. Then I must thank Rebecca Claire for encouraging me to tape hours and hours of my life and Pagan for transcribing the hours and hours of tapes into print. Michelle Meizner, thank you for being the loving interpreter of my tired, slurred speech from tape to computer. I will always adore you, Clove Tsindle, for being an incessant nag, asking loving questions upon loving questions to deepen and strengthen the feeling of this book, and just because you're you. Thanks to Maryanne Smith for buying me a voice activated tape recorder so I could be alone to tape the more intimate parts of my story.

My heartfelt respect and appreciation goes to the numerous personal care assistants (PCAs) I have had throughout the twelve years that it took to bring the dream of this book into reality. They were the ones who had to awaken at four in the morning to write down that perfect phrase, stay up with me till three while I had to finish a chapter, or get me up and dressed really early in the morning after I had been up late the night before because my transcriber was coming. They gave of their sleep, their strength and of their quiet non-intrusive respect for my floundering with words as they erased, wrote, crossed out, wrote and erased again my many corrections and changes. It was not an easy task to find the right word on the page, directed only by my eyes and voice.

Su Flickinger gave of herself first as a PCA, then as a transcriber and also as a mentor. She never stopped believing in me and the message I had to share. I bless her for that. I thank you, Nina Brand, for helping me send out many manuscripts. Thanks to Irv Zola for his expertise in editing for ableist language and his detailed support in contract for-mulation. I'm also grateful to Paul Fitzgerald for creative edi-torial feedback. I wish to thank Rachel Lebowitz, my most recent "find." She has been an accurate, diligent and pushy-when-necessary transcriber who has kept the thousands of pages, copies, copyeditor's notes and my editor's notes all straight.

I am eternally grateful to Marge Schneider, from Women's Braille Press, who helped me find a publisher sensitive to the issues at hand. Holly Morris, my editor from Seal Press, has been the perfect editor—patient, responsible, thoughtful, caring and competent. I thank her especially for her non-threatening, never-in-a-hurry attitude.

I wish to express my love and appreciation to Charlotte Podalsky, my first, last, and forever therapist and friend who was always there when I needed her. Heartfelt thanks to Doctors Dale Weldon and Mark Johnson for keeping me alive through high-risk, life-saving surgery that other doc-tors refused to attempt. They knew that I had to survive at least long enough to finish *The Me in the Mirror*.

Words cannot express all that Ron Kovic gave me and taught me about how to write a book. He always knew that I had to write one. His feedback and encouragement were invaluable—not necessarily in the roughest parts of the jour-ney, but often in the long quiet stretches when I forgot I had to keep writing.

Of course I want to say thank you to all my friends—Janet Bernault, John Kelly, Cindy Miller, Arachne Stevens, Kay Hagemann, Kady, Janet Pearl, Bill Eyman, Nova Robinson, Dorothy Baronholtz, Kelley Ellsworth, Mary Stockton, Margo Richard, Chrystos, Jennifer Justice, Joyce Garber and Lou Krodel—who stood, sat and lay by me with comfort, encouragement, and humor, cheering me on day and night, in person, by phone and by letter, until I completed my story. I remember with special gratitude the love and energy given by the late Terry Smith, John Gallant and my grandmother. I know they must be smiling proudly at me at this moment.

And of course, thanks to Dianna, my cat, for providing the very important "time-outs." Just before I got too tired to think, she would plop down in the middle of the manuscript and purr loudly.

And finally thanks to my lover, Judy Brewer, who continues to ride the ups and downs of my menopause, and my ever changing disability along with the ups and downs of my writing. It was Judy who stayed up late into the night printing copy after copy on her printer. She often gave me feedback lovingly in the face of fierce indignation. It was Judy who held me through tears and fears, and laughed and danced with me in celebration after each hurdle. Judy's loving and challenging feedback allowed me to grow in my writing and surpass myself.

CONTENTS

INTRODUCTION

When you are disabled, some people look to you for wis-
dom, others look at you in fear; most of the world doesn't
notice you or tries not to. And in the midst of all their con-
ceptions of you, you exist. You are yourself, alone with your
pain, your guilt, your own terror. No one can ever get inside
your body to understand what it's like. Being disabled, you
find yourself alone in your joy as well. You experience great
victories too small for most able-bodied to notice.

For many years I have pondered how to write about my
"exceptional" life without sounding pompous, crazy or
preachy. I don't want to increase able-bodied guilt. I want to
write for my disabled sisters, for my disabled brothers and,
still, I am concerned with how the able-bodied will react because they will take that reaction out into the world with
them. My words may either enable them to see every being
as divinely unique and different, or my words may challenge
them too much. If I dare challenge the reality of the able too
much, they may unknowingly or otherwise inflict more grief
upon those of us who struggle daily with the oppression of
being different.

I write the following words out of love for the breath of
life which is so very precious to me and for love of changing
the world. I write for all the mothers and fathers and sisters
and brothers of people with disabilities. They have shared
the oppression, the inaccessibility, and the pain that we go
through every day. I write so that personal assistance and
universal accessibility become realities. If at times my words
seem angry, if they sound resentful or confused, they still
come from a loving place in my heart.

ON DISABLED CHILDREN

Don't rip these children
from their wombs
merely because they have no limbs
with which to grasp

Blind eyes plead
not to be destroyed
like the broken toys
the Nazis cooked
to perfect the master race

Connie Panzarino

I

CLAY PIE

In the art room of the Human Resources Center, I watched Eddie make a clay pie similar to those he made week after week. He cut it in half, saying, "I don't want this part, that's the yucky part."

I responded, "That's okay, I'll take that part."

He took the piece of clay in his right hand and stood up. With his left hand dangling at his side, he pressed the piece into my right hand. "You can't use that hand?" he questioned me, pointing to my left hand.

"No, I don't use it a lot, but I can hold things in it. I like the way it looks and the way it feels."

Eddie sat down and looked at his paralyzed left arm. He looked again at mine. With his right hand, he lifted his left arm up onto the table, onto his half clay pie, and used his right hand to cut the pie.

I asked, "You can hold things with your left hand too, can't you?"

Eddie smiled and handed a piece of his pie to Maggie, my attendant, with his left hand. That was the first time this five-year-old boy with cerebral palsy had willingly used his left arm. I noticed he stopped cutting the "yucky" part off of all his clay pieces from that point on.

"We have to clean up now," I said at the end of the hour. "Maggie, will you help Eddie put the clay away and wash

3

up?" She nodded and helped Eddie wash up. "I'll walk Eddie back to his class. Can you gather our things together and meet me at the van?" She nodded.

"Open the van, Mag," I called, speeding along the sidewalk. I zipped onto the lift. Maggie worked the switches which lifted me up into the van. I rolled in, positioned myself between the front seats and nodded to Maggie. On my cue, she put on the straps that held the chair in place, turned my chair off, and put on my seatbelt. Maggie and I drove from the Human Resources Center to my dorm at New York University. "Step on it," I directed her, "I have to go to the bathroom, eat and get to class in two hours." As she accelerated I cautioned her, "Don't go over ninety."

About ten minutes later, we heard a siren. Maggie moaned, "Damn, Connie, it's a cop."

"Quick! Get off at the next exit. Pull in that gas station, open the hood and pretend there's something wrong with the engine."

As Maggie was standing with her head under the hood, a cop got out of his car and asked her for her license and registration. She waved him off and told him to wait. She closed the hood and came into the van, turning first to the officer and telling him to wait just one more minute, she'd be right with him.

I whispered, "Quick, my meds."

Maggie pulled out a vial of my pills, put one in my mouth, and got my cup of water out from under my electric wheelchair. She poked her head out the window and said, "Sorry, Officer, I had to give this woman her medication, how can I help you?"

The officer stuttered, "Do you know how fast you were going?"

"No, Officer, how fast were we going?" Maggie asked as I chewed up my pills and asked her for a sip.

Maggie turned away from the officer, gave me my sip and looked back at him. "Eighty miles an hour!" he said.

"Yes," I said. "We were having engine trouble and I had to take medication and I figured It would be safer to hurry up and get to a gas station. Maggie, let me have another pill. Excuse me, Officer," I took a sip and swallowed.

Maggie said, "I looked under the hood but everything seemed to be okay. Officer, do you want to take a look?"

The officer just frowned and said that Maggie wasn't supposed to speed around like that, especially with people like me in the van. "What would your boss say if I told him?" he asked.

"She's my boss." Maggie pointed to me. "This is her van."

I smiled at the officer. He tossed his hands in the air, shook his head, and told us if we wanted to live longer, we should slow down; and that if you have engine trouble, you're not supposed to speed up. He went away mumbling and drove off. We waited until he was out of sight and took off again.

"We're doing eighty-five," Maggie said.

"Good," I said, "I have to go to the bathroom really bad."

As we approached the Weinstein dorm on University Place, I directed Maggie in parallel parking. I told her to unstrap my chair, turn it on, and instructed her in positioning my hand so I could drive the chair. She opened the lift, and I descended to the sidewalk. She closed up the van and walked with me up the street to the ramp while passersby had various reactions ranging from smiling and nodding, staring, or turning their heads, to bumping into my chair and apologizing profusely, as if they had caused my condition.

"Any messages?" I asked, passing the front desk as Maggie checked my mailbox.

"There's one from your attorney about your court date and one from a new attendant applicant." Maggie held open the elevator door as she leafed through my mail.

"Open the lights, get the bedpan and hand me the phone," I directed her as I parked my chair alongside the bed. Maggie handed me the phone and braced my hand against the receiver so it wouldn't slip. "Dial Mr. Brewer."

My attorney, Curtis Brewer, informed me that after seven years, we finally had a court date. Perhaps, I thought, by the time I finish this Master's program at age thirty-three, I will actually be allowed to work legally. I raised my eyebrows at Maggie, looking from the receiver to the phone, to signal her to hang up.

I nodded to Maggie and she removed the armrest from my chair as well as my safety belt. "Take off the foot pedals," I said. She lifted my feet to the floor. I began slowly swinging my legs one inch in either direction while singing, "Zippity doo dah." It took all my might, but it felt good. Maggie laughed. "Okay," I said, "Let's go." She lifted me on to the bed. She pulled my pants down, rolled me over and positioned me on the bedpan. When I said "I'm done," she rolled me over, wiped me, pulled up my pants, straightened my clothes and lifted me back into the chair.

Maggie emptied the bedpan and used the bathroom herself while I made mental notes of what we needed to take. When she came back, I said, "Let me call in my case notes, and while I'm doing that, get my two notebooks, my art therapy text book by Edith Kramer and my jacket." Maggie propped the phone against me and dialed Dorothy's number so I could leave my case notes on her answering machine for her to transcribe that evening. I needed to present them in seminar the next morning.

"Open the door," I said, and whizzed down the hall with Maggie close at my wheels. "Did you lock the door?" I asked.

"Oops!" she exclaimed as she ran back to lock the door.

We took the elevator to the basement and got in the cafeteria line. It was crowded. People started tripping over me, and telling me to go to the head of the line, which I immediately did since I was in a hurry and figured they would feel good about helping the handicapped.

Choosing dinner was a real challenge since I could no longer chew and swallow tough things like salad or meat, couldn't eat hot spicy foods because of my ulcer and because I was trying to avoid sugar. They had leather-like roast beef, mashed potatoes, (which I could eat), Mexican bean loaf and barbequed chicken wings. I asked for mashed potatoes and gravy and told Maggie to get me some cottage cheese from the salad bar. I also asked for applesauce, which was probably sweetened with sugar, but I couldn't figure out anything else to eat. The guy behind the counter ignored me. People kept going around me in line. I shouted at the guy several times, but he didn't pay attention until one of the passing students told him to serve me. The student put my dinner on my laptray.

We got to the checkout and I had Maggie show the woman my ID, entitling me to dinner. She told me that Maggie wasn't allowed to sit with me or eat the food unless she paid $3.75. I was in a rush, and this was a new cashier. I explained politely that Maggie had to feed me, that she was my attendant and had brought her own food. Maggie waved her brown paper bag in front of the woman and offered to show her her dinner. The woman was adamant that we follow the rules. I told her she should call the manager and pressed on past her. Maggie followed, grabbed silverware and sat down. On cue from me she began feeding me and eating her sandwich. I still preferred to feed myself, but it took so much energy and too much time. I needed to save my hand strength for class.

"Good thing you took your pills in the van," she said, "we only have fifteen minutes to eat."

"Yep," I said, with a mouthful of mashed potatoes. I knew I couldn't eat very much in fifteen minutes without choking, so I asked Maggie to run back and grab me a milk so I could drink some fast protein. As she left, the manager appeared and asked me what the problem was. I reminded him that there was no problem as long as he told the cashier that I had permission to have my attendants here. I told him that nothing had changed since last week or the two weeks before that, and that I still needed someone to feed me.

"Well, if you just had one attendant the whole time, we could give her an ID with a picture on it. Then there wouldn't be any problem," he said.

"Well, if you just had one cashier all the time, she would know I always have an attendant and there wouldn't be any problem. You need many cashiers and I need many attendants."

He left. I saw him talking to the cashier and pointing at me.

Maggie came back and I drank half the milk. "I don't want to drink too much 'cause I can't go to the bathroom until we get back to the dorm tonight, and I won't make it until then. Can you get the hair out of my eyes? Thanks."

Maggie helped me put my jacket on and we left for my "Art for the Art Therapist" class. When we got there, the elevator was stuck and wouldn't come. Maggie ran upstairs to see if she could find it. It was on the third floor. Someone had switched it off. She turned it on and rode it to the first floor. I got on and we arrived in class on time.

Maggie turned on my pocket tape recorder for the first twenty minutes of lecture time in class. Then she helped position my hand to hold the paint brush that we were using for the class exercise. Since I could cover only about a four-inch-span, I often directed her with my eyes and occasional whispers to move the paper left, right, up or down. We were painting "feeling small." The exercise was fun, but quite fatiguing. Several times I found myself panting from the effort and would need to stop and rest.

One of the other students offered to put my work up on the board with hers.

The professor, Edith Kramer, told us, "Take a break and look at each other's work. We will reconvene in fifteen minutes."

I moved a few of the chairs out of the way by pushing them with my wheelchair. I tried guessing whose work was whose by their style and subject matter.

Allison asked, "Connie, do you want a cup of coffee? I'm going over to the deli."

"Can you get me a yogurt? I'm starving. Maggie, give Allison some money from my wallet. Do you want anything, Maggie?"

"Yeah, I'd love a cup of coffee."

"Allison, do you mind getting Maggie a cup of coffee also?"

"Nope. Be right back. What do you take in it, Maggie?"

"Just cream. Thanks."

"Jean," I said, "how's your placement going?"

"Better," she said. "I think the patients are beginning to trust me. How's your placement?"

"Great, except I wish the staff was as comfortable with me as the kids are. How was your weekend?"

"Pretty good. Worked a lot. Had company Sunday."

"I played more than I worked this weekend. Couldn't resist the beautiful weather," I said.

Allison came back with the yogurt and coffee. The class gathered for discussion. Maggie fed me my yogurt, trying to space the spoonfuls between the discussion.

We left class and as we walked along the street, my hand began to grow numb from the cold. "It's too cold, Mag, I can't drive any more." She took over the joystick and steered my chair shakily back to the dorm. We went up to my room and I read my notes for the next day while Maggie took a shower.

"Set up the respirator, get the meds and the bedpan." As she did I thought about what to wear the next day. "Start giving me my pills and take out my brown pants, blue sweater and the silk scarf that goes with them. I'll wear my sneakers. Take out underwear."

After taking my pills, Maggie undressed me, lifted me up

on the bed, helped me use the bedpan, positioned me under the covers and set me up with the respirator for a half-hour treatment. "Boy, am I congested tonight!" I mumbled with the respirator in my mouth. "Too much dairy." As I finished my treatment, Maggie straightened up the room. "I'm done breathing."

She smiled and took the respirator out of my mouth. "Ready to turn?"

"Yeah, I'm beat."

Maggie turned me on my side and positioned my arms and legs so that there would be the least pressure to cause sores or pain during the night. She put tissues under my cheek so I could spit or dribble to avoid choking. She washed the respirator, charged my electric wheelchair, turned out the light and went to bed.

Two hours later I called out, "Maggie, turn me."

Maggie stumbled over to me in her half-sleep, pulled the covers back, threw the tissues away, turned me, repositioned new tissues, covered me and stumbled back to bed. This happened twice more before morning.

The alarm went off at seven A.M. "Maggie. Maggie! The alarm."

Maggie got up and turned off the alarm. She set up the respirator and put me on it. She went to get dressed, made her bed, and got the chair ready. She brought the bedpan and a basin of hot water. Soon I told her, "I'm done." She took the respirator away and washed it.

"Wash my face." Taking cues and directions from me, Maggie washed me up, helped me use the bedpan and dressed me for the day. When I was ready she lifted me into my chair. "Brush my teeth and then comb my hair." There was a knock at the door. "Oh no, it's eight o'clock already!"

Janet came in for her shift. She put her things away and finished brushing my hair as Maggie collected her things and got ready to leave.

"See ya all next week," Maggie said.

"Take care, thanks a lot, Mag."

"Bye, Maggie," said Janet.

Janet and I went down to the cafeteria to get my break-fast. Rubbery, unswallowable eggs again. "I'll take yogurt and toast."

When we got up to the lobby of the dorm, it was pouring. "Damn! Can you drive the van up front?" I asked Janet.

"I'll try, boss!" she said, goofing on me.

She put my rain poncho on me and left. People were staring at me—students, teachers, a babe in arms. I looked very weird. I smiled, sheepishly. I knew I looked odd with this bright orange poncho draped over me and my entire chair. It was also warm. Janet pulled up in front of the dorm. As I moved towards the door, the security guard offered to open it for me. I thanked him and raced out into the rain and onto the van lift. My electric wheelchair always hated rain, and so it temporarily stalled. It took me a few minutes to position myself in the van.

We crowded into the seminar. The room was made for three and there were six of us. One by one we presented and discussed our case material.

Mary, who worked at the hospital school for delinquent boys, said, "J.R. is a sixteen-year-old boy diagnosed with paranoid schizophrenia. He has been hospitalized for eight months. I've been working with him for the past six weeks. He was referred to me because he was not verbalizing his feelings with his psychologist. He is withdrawn, but compliant. I have here three of the drawings he has done in the last two sessions." The pictures depicted nude women.

Jackie said, "Well, he has a healthy libido."

"I know," agreed Mary, "but I think I'm a little afraid of that. He has begun to ask me if I like going out to dinner or dancing, and I'm afraid he's going to get a crush on me and ask me out."

Allison pointed out, "That's normal, though, isn't it? I mean, kids get crushes on their teachers all the time."

"Yeah," I said, "and as long as you take it as a compliment while still refusing, he should be okay."

"Still, I understand why Mary would be concerned because this is not a normal sixteen-year-old, and she doesn't want to cause him any more pain than he already has," said Jackie.

I noticed that Mary was very well dressed, with a tight skirt, low-cut blouse, lots of makeup and jewelry. "Mary, do you dress similarly at work to what you're wearing here?"

"Well, yes. The materials we use aren't really that messy, and I have to represent cases at staff meetings. I want to appear as professional as possible."

"It would be better for your client at his vulnerable age, and also more practical for you, to consider wearing a smock while you're in the art room," suggested Professor Kramer. "I never had too many of those problems because I'm older so I'm more like a mother or grandmother."

Bea presented the case of S.P., her client, a blind nine-year-old boy who was acting out in class. He was referred to art therapy because he was angry, hitting other children and doing poorly in his studies. His parents were divorced. He spent weekends with his father. He had six siblings, two sisters and four brothers. He was the youngest child.

"He can't seem to finish a project. We worked with clay, and he started making a car and then tore it up. He wanted to paint. I told him which colors were which and he painted a house but never finished the roof. I've brought in some of his partial sculptures. They're very regressive. I can't tell if he's angry at being blind—I mean, he must be. I just don't know how to interpret his work," said Bea.

Edith said, "Well, I can tell you I do not think this is just about disability. I mean after all, look at Connie's art work. She is obviously a well-adjusted disabled person who must have had a loving, warm family and a fairly normal childhood to produce such integrated and grounded artwork. This child, S.P., has many other family problems in his life."

Bea asked, "What do you think, Connie?"

"I think. . . I don't know," I replied, and sank into a fog of childhood memories.

2

GREEN WALLS

My parents said that as an infant I was an active, good baby who slept well and delighted all the relatives. When I was seven months old, they said that I couldn't pull myself into a sitting position and could not maintain my head and neck balance the way other children did. I never crawled. I was different, but no one knew what was "wrong" with me. Soon after began years of doctors, medicines and expensive treatments and there was never enough money to pay for them.

As far back as I remember there were many trips to the doctors. They were dreadful, and they were all so far away. I wondered why the doctors didn't want to live near us. I remember the long rides in the car, sitting between my parents. I couldn't see anything but the tops of trees, telephone poles and every once in a while a bird or plane that would fly over. My parents were tense and quiet. The rides were mostly boring, but I could never seem to drift off to sleep. The pit of my stomach ached too much.

All the doctors had green rooms. I don't know whether it was the color-of-the-year, cheap World War II surplus paint, or whatever, but I remember green—lots of it. It was a sickening grayish-green. I have vivid memories of different colored examination tables—green, maroon, brown—all of them padded with plastic, but the tables still felt hard. Many of them were covered with paper, which made crinkly

14

noises and caused me to slip very easily. One time when I started to slip I couldn't stop myself. My mother grabbed me just in time.

The exams themselves felt dangerous. I was always naked and cold. They probed and whispered. Being high up on a table, four feet off the ground, felt scary. I was always afraid of falling, and I would exhaust myself at each appointment trying to hold my balance. Since I had so little strength, I held myself up on the table by balancing. I would prop myself up on my elbow or lean my shoulder against my mother. Move me too fast and I'd fall. I couldn't stay in one position too long without my muscles fatiguing.

I was asked to do all the kinds of things I couldn't do—lift my head, move my arm, move my foot—and of course I failed, over and over again. I felt bad that I couldn't do what was being asked of me. After all, who would ask a child to do something they couldn't do? I thought I should be able to do normal things like other children, since I looked and felt like them. Nobody seemed to care that at ten months I was able to talk. Perhaps because I could speak, or because these visits were so tortuous, I have clear memories of them.

The doctors seemed crazy, putting me through tortures like banging me with little hammers, sticking me with safety pins to see if I could feel, and taking parts of me for lab tests. So when I was a year old and all these different doctors, nurses and people in white jackets couldn't find anything wrong, I figured I had passed the test and nothing was wrong with me. I just couldn't walk.

"Mommy, I want to go home."

"Shh! So, what do you think, Doctor?"

"Well, Mrs. Panzarino, in these cases time can tell a lot, but there's no evidence of the common diseases. The muscle biopsy we did five months ago was negative. Are you feeding her well?"

My father said, "She seems to drink her bottle and eat some, how much can a fourteen-month-old eat?"

"Well, Mr. Panzarino, do you allow your daughter to get exercise? I mean, little children need to run around, play."

"Doctor, that's why we're here. She can't run around. She can't even stand, you saw that for yourself. What's wrong with her?" asked my mother.

"Mr. and Mrs. Panzarino, her reflexes are fine. She may grow out of it. She's very healthy. I don't know what more you want from me at this time. If you like, you can come back in six months or a year and we'll talk again," said the doctor.

"Mommy, you okay?"

My mother didn't answer me. She began to dress me silently. She rubbed over the biopsy scar that ran from my right hip to right knee, and frowned. I thought she was upset.

The drive home always had an air of despair. My parents were let down and tired. I was tired, too. The tension had been replaced by disappointment because we had gotten the bad news again that there was no news, that nothing was wrong with me. I used to think maybe I *should* have something wrong with me. I bit my arms to relieve my frustration. It left marks like the one on the side of my leg. Maybe if I bit myself hard enough they would finally find something wrong.

My diet was always changing, so I never knew what I could eat. Some of the doctors made me try salt-free diets and others insisted on salty ones. Friends advised my mother to feed me vitamin cocktails. I couldn't have ice cream and candy bars like the rest of the kids. They were eating candy bars and walking. I was drinking carrot juice and being carried.

• • •

When I was two, a physical therapist named Miss Midwood came to the house twice a week to show my mother how to do therapy with me. I liked her. I didn't like the exercises. I would have to lie on the kitchen table and be stretched, and once again, I was told to do all kinds of things I couldn't do. It was painful and sometimes I cried. She gave me a book depicting God as a warm, fatherly person. It made me feel better somehow. She also tried to make me feel better by telling me that if I couldn't do something then, that I might be able to do it later. She was the only person that ever said that to me. It felt good to hear that, but I didn't believe her. I just smiled.

I felt really uncomfortable sitting at kitchen tables. How could I eat at the same table where somebody exercised me? There were other tortures that made me uncomfortable in that kitchen.

There was an exercise I had to do in the two kitchen sinks. One sink was filled with very hot water and the other with cold. My mother would sit me on the edge between the two and alternate putting my feet in each sink. First, she plunged them into the hot water for a couple of minutes, then into the cold water, back and forth repeatedly. It was supposed to improve my circulation, but it felt like hell. It shocked my whole body. My mother said it wasn't painful, and then got mad at me when I cried.

One day, my mother sat me at my little table in the living room to play. My feet dangled in toe-down position.

"Keep your feet up on this book. The doctor said not to let your feet hang down, otherwise we won't be able to get rid of those contractions," she directed as she bent my knees up and placed my feet flat on a big fat yellow phone book.

"It hurts!"

"It doesn't hurt that much. Besides, you need to get your

feet straightened out or you'll never walk."

She gave me a hug and went in the kitchen to do dishes. I concentrated hard and struggled until I slid my feet off the telephone book.

The doorbell rang. It was the insurance man. He came in to collect payments from my mother, saw me at my table, and said, "Oh! Hi, how are you? Are you being a good girl today?"

I nodded yes.

My mother said, "No, she's not. Look at her feet. They're on the floor again. I keep putting her feet on books so they won't dangle. We don't want her to have contractions. She's supposed to keep her feet up on that thing."

I looked at him a little sheepishly.

He said, "You be a good girl. You should keep your feet up on the book like your mother tells you, otherwise how are you gonna walk?"

I gave him a dirty look, thinking to myself, "Who's gonna walk?"

He said, "You know someday you might walk, and then if your feet are bent, you won't be able to do anything about it."

I looked him dead in the eye and said, "I'll be a ballerina and I'll walk on my toes."

Aunt Kay married a young man named Anthony. He became my new uncle. I loved him. He had a lot of energy and would sing songs with me. I couldn't say Anthony right when I was very young, although I didn't seem to have trouble with any other words. "Anthony" somehow came out "Eckie."

I would be waiting for him when he came home from work, and when I saw him coming down the block, I'd yell, "Eckie!" He would yell back, "Connie!" and we would continue yelling back and forth. It was my way of running to meet him.

The Christmas I was three, I got a big present. Mommy and Daddy helped me open it. I couldn't unwrap presents by myself, though I would try by biting and tearing the ribbons with my teeth. It was a rocking horse from Santa. Even Santa wanted me to be normal. For months I tried so hard to keep my balance on that dumb horse. By spring, I wanted to throw it out our second-story window, only I didn't want to seem ungrateful. They were trying to help me use a toy that any of my cousins or friends would have loved. We kept it around for years. Every once in a while I would sit on it, but I was never able to ride it.

One afternoon when I was about four, I was sitting as usual at my little table playing. Mom was busy cleaning I was coloring and dropped the red crayon. I finished most of the picture without using red, but now it was time to color the lips of the little girl in the picture.

"Mom!" I called.

"Just a minute," she answered.

I slid one foot off the telephone book and took all the crayons out of the box and put them in a neat row according to color.

"Mom!" I called again. "I need the crayon I dropped."

Mom came in, picked up the crayon, looked at the picture I colored, and smiled. "That's beautiful, honey. Do you want to do more coloring, or do you want me to get you something else to play with?"

"I'll color. Can I have my ball?"

Mom found my ball and put it in my hands saying, "Now don't drop it, okay? Mommy's got a lot of work to do." She kissed me on the cheek and walked out of the room.

I leaned forward over the table and tucked the ball under

my chest while I colored the lips red. I wiggled my other foot off the book onto the floor. What a relief. I printed my name at the bottom of the picture and started another one. My hand started to get tired. I had short sleeves on and my arms stuck to the table making me feel fat, like the Pillsbury Doughboy. I couldn't slide my arms to get the crayons the way I usually did when I had on long sleeves, so I took hold of my right thumb with my teeth, arched my head back, and lifted my arm like a crane, my teeth being the jaws.

I began bouncing the ball about four inches high on the table, catching it in my hands and rolling it back and forth. I imagined running and playing like my cousins did. As my fantasy grew, so did the arc that the ball was traveling in. Finally, I lost it over the edge of the table. "Mom!" I shouted.

She ran in, "What happened?"

I looked at her wide-eyed in fear, saying, "I dropped my ball."

She looked annoyed, but picked it up and gave it back to me. She warned me that she was not going to come in every time I dropped the ball. "If you want to play with it, don't throw it. Do you want anything else?"

"No," I said, sulking.

She went back to her chores and I began studying the furniture in the living room. Right across from me there was a credenza. It was a big piece of furniture with large drawers and cabinets and glass shelves on either side. The shelves had figurines on them, and behind the shelves there were mirrors. I sat across from one of them.

There was another "Connie" in the mirror. I noticed that she was looking sad like me. I smiled, and she smiled back.

I was lonely, so I decided to talk to the other Connie. "Hi," I whispered and then waved. She waved back.

"Why don't you come over here and dance with me on my side of the mirror? It's nice over here," she said.

"No, I can't. You come over here," I whispered. "We can play ball."

"No, I don't want to. Why can't you come here?" she said.

"Because I can't walk," I said.

The other Connie replied, "Sure you can. If *I* can, *you* can. Come on over."

I looked at her sitting happily across from me. She looked like the pictures taken of me at Christmas and on my birthday that were in Mommy's photo albums. I was always sitting in them. But the Connie in the pictures didn't move, and the Connie in the mirror could.

"You don't like me," she said, "otherwise you'd come and play with me."

"No, I do like you," I said softly. "I just can't walk."

"Yes, you can," she retorted.

"No, I can't!" I shouted.

"What?" my mother yelled from another room.

"Nothing!" I shouted to my mother. "Be quiet," I whispered to the other Connie.

"How do you know you can't walk?" Connie asked.

"Because that's what Mommy told the doctors," I said.

"Did you ever try?"

"No," I whimpered, "I'll fall."

I threw my ball at the other Connie in the mirror and said, "Catch."

She didn't catch it and scowled back at me.

My mother appeared from nowhere saying, "Who were you talking to? Why aren't your feet on the book? I told you not to throw the ball. Can't you be good?"

She put my feet roughly back on the book and turned to a clean coloring page. "Color," she said. She put the ball away and brought out three Little Golden books for me to read and put them within my reach.

I picked up a book and leafed through three or four pages. "Mom," I called. "I have to go to the bathroom."

A response came from the other room. "You wait. I was just in there. Why didn't you tell me then? Now I'm in the middle of something. You wait."

I began rocking to ease the discomfort. My feet were hurting from being up on the book, but I was afraid to wiggle them off. I began to squeeze my thighs together. That always felt good and took my mind off my bladder for a while. Every few minutes I would stop rocking and call out, "Mom, I can't wait."

She would either not answer or warn me with, "Don't make me come in there before I'm ready."

Suddenly in the midst of my rocking, she appeared, snapping, "I know what you're doing, you stop that business."

She picked me up over her shoulder and carried me into the bathroom. She pulled down my pants and held me on the toilet until I got my balance. It was very hard for me to balance. I remember once my father had put me on the toilet and walked away fast. I fell on my head. Mom was much more careful about things like that, even when she was tired and rushed.

When I was done, she picked me up over her shoulder, wiped me, and pulled my pants up. "Where do you want to sit?" she asked.

"In the kitchen with you," I said.

"You can't, I just washed the floor. Why don't you sit on the couch and play with your dolls?" she said, putting me on the couch. She gave me my dolls and asked, "Do you want anything else now? I have to go clean the bathroom."

"No," I said, and smiled up at her. She walked away.

It was tiring to play with most toys because I was so weak. Lifting a wooden block was like lifting a cement block, and my baby doll was as heavy to me as a real infant. I would pant and sweat just to lift her to my shoulder to burp her.

Many people thought the struggling was good for me and would avert their eyes. They seemed to think if I worked hard enough I would build up my muscles and be fine. I didn't want to be a weightlifter, just a ballerina! The only thing the straining ever did for me was make me want to give up and recede into myself. When this happened, parents, adult relatives and their friends would shock me back into reality with a sharp word or light slap. I would feel angry and invaded.

My grandmother, though, was different. When she saw me struggling with my toys, she would help me. When I stared blankly into space, she would approach me gently with a kiss or caress, candy or food treat, or singsong my name or some endearing expression. Having gotten my attention, she would then play a while with me.

Grandma always put things near enough so I could get them easily instead of making me reach out and strain myself. She always cut my food small enough for me to eat safely. When food was too big, especially meat, sometimes I choked on it until I turned blue.

I think my grandmother understood how hard it was. Even trying to do simple things for myself was a daily struggle. Grandma knew I escaped into fantasy. She knew that unless there were things for me to enjoy in the world around me, I would not stay in the present. It was maddening to be so immobile. I don't know what she thought about my condition, but I know she loved me.

I didn't have many playmates back then, but those I had were special, like my cousin Vinny. He was a year younger than me. He would dance with me. If I was crying he would come over and put his face real close to mine, look me seriously in the eye, and ask if I was okay. Sometimes he would perform silly antics to make me laugh. He whispered secrets to me, like what goodies he saw in the refrigerator or pantry. We were both chubby, food-loving children. He loved animals and shared that joy with me by bringing over various neighborhood pets to meet me.

Vinny also teased me. I think part of the reason behind

the teasing was that he wanted me to be normal. One day, while we played under the grapevine in my grandmother's backyard, we decided we were going to make wine. Though we weren't allowed to watch grandpa make wine, we had often watched grandma make grape jelly, and we figured the process couldn't be that different. We put a bunch of grapes in a pot, and Vinny smashed them with rocks, making a grand old mess. He stuck his hands in, squeezing and squirting the grapes while I lustily cheered him on.

"I'm gonna get you!" he said, raising his purple, dripping hands up to my face.

I screamed and felt the urge to slap his hands away, but I knew I wasn't fast enough, so I screamed again, "No! Stop it!"

He laughed, and I would have too, if I wasn't so terrified that the grape juice would drip on my clothes and my mother would get mad.

My screams eventually brought Aunt Ro to the door yelling, "Stop that, Vinny! Don't you know she can't fight back? God's gonna punish you! Now don't you make me come out there."

Another favorite game was to slap me on my legs or arms, and run. At first he would look back expectantly, waiting for me to chase him. After a while he realized I couldn't, so that became the game. He would grab my doll, or any toy I happened to be playing with, and prance around with it just out of my reach. I hated it, yet felt somehow accepted by him because the teasing was the same kind of attention that other little girls got from little boys.

Sometimes we were pals and would get into trouble together. Once in a while, Vinny was downright sensitive, bringing me a flower from the garden, or sharing a new toy, but teasing was his favorite pastime.

Though it made me angry at the time, I think I needed someone to be angry at. It gave me a safe outlet through which to focus and express the rage I felt at not being able to move. We played this game where we would sit real close together, close our eyes, and bang our foreheads together as hard as we could until we got dizzy. Then we would laugh hysterically. A few times Aunt Ro caught us and yelled at us, "Stop that! You're going to make yourself stupid."

My mother's cousin, Gloria, lived upstairs in my grandmother's house. She wasn't quite an adult, but she was bigger than us kids. We could be alone with her on the front stoop and not have to have an adult there. It felt nicer than being with the adults and you could talk about what you wanted to. She didn't like boys, and she thought I was wonderful. She didn't seem to be uncomfortable when I couldn't do what the other kids did. She even helped my mother take care of me once in a while. She was very determined and strong, and I wanted to grow up to be just like her. I liked that she wasn't particularly "pretty," the way other kids in the family were thought to be pretty. I thought she was beautiful. She held herself tall and looked directly at you. She had presence, and was forceful but not overbearing.

There were a lot of things I couldn't do, even though I looked fine. I couldn't open jars and boxes, but then, I was a kid, and most kids needed help with those things. I couldn't cut my meat or even swallow it very well. I couldn't dress myself or turn over in bed. I had to be moved and handled in much the same way people handle infants. My neck had to be supported at all times. I had to be laid down and rolled over to put my pants on.

As I got bigger, the movements became more difficult. I couldn't sit up and when someone pushed a shirt over my head the way you would with a toddler, I would fall over backwards. My mother encouraged me to help her dress me. She would ask me to try to put my arm in the sleeve, but most of the time I couldn't really do it, and it just made me tired. I attempted to move my body with her, rather than fighting her movements or just going limp. We became a team very early on, at least at dressing.

I loved playing with Tinkertoys, but I couldn't push them together hard enough to connect them well. To pull them apart, I would grab the top with my teeth. To put the stick in the hole I would lean on it with my head to push it down. I used my teeth, head and chin a lot when I played. Most of the things I made fell apart.

If my mother didn't use a baby carriage to get me around, I was carried. People would often stare at me, or ask my mother a lot of questions because I was obviously too big to be in a baby carriage or in someone's arms. We lived on the second floor of a walk-up in Brooklyn, so I had to be carried up and down the stairs. My father did that as well as most of the long-distance carrying. Not only was he a lot stronger, he was rougher. He wasn't always aware of how much work it was for me to balance myself. It was hard to keep my equilibrium in somebody's arms while they were moving, especially if they were going downstairs. If they weren't aware of the need to steady me I would get really exhausted and feel like I was falling—just like when I was on the examination table.

When I got tired and complained, my father would say impatiently, "What's the matter?" He didn't realize what he was doing, or rather not doing, but to me it was like riding a horse. Even though my father was stronger, my mother really knew how to support my back and hips and aid my balance.

It was terrible to be in a limbo of having something wrong with me and feeling like there was nothing wrong with me. I hated not being able to do things other people could do and not knowing what that meant. I couldn't begin to define myself because I was not like others around me, yet I felt like them.

Sometimes I was treated like everyone else. "Okay, you

kids. It's time for bed, now," Aunt Ro would shout. Vinny and I would whine and beg to stay up, but invariably we would get carted off to bed.

Other times, I was treated differently. Mom would come out and put a jacket and hat on me because she said it was cold, even though Vinny was running around in shirt sleeves.

"I don't want a jacket," I whined, knowing that I couldn't move as well with heavier clothing. "How come he doesn't have to put one on?"

"Never mind him," retorted Mom.

I developed the illusion that everybody else was weird and that I was fine. The illusion worked for a while, but obviously most people were walking, and most kids could do things I couldn't do. So who was the weird one? I remember pushing the thoughts away because they felt dangerous. If I dug too deeply I might shatter the illusion and be left with the reality that something terrible was wrong with me. Something that no one could name, let alone fix. Being other than "normal" made me feel like a blown-glass figure that people kept on their coffee tables to look at but that no one was supposed to touch.

If I wanted to play a game with the other kids, like hide-and-seek, I would ask my mother, "Can I play hide-and-seek?" I would get very confused when she'd say, "No, you can't play that game." I imagined I could hide, even though somebody would have to hide me. Actually, if they found me, I wouldn't have been able to come out, and I also couldn't find the other people who were hiding. It was so confusing.

Sometimes I'd get mad at Mom; sometimes I'd just feel sad. I wasn't sure if it was Mom's fault that I couldn't play a game because she wouldn't let me play, or if she was merely showing me the reality that I was not able to play. Once, I wanted her to buy me a jump rope. I told her if I couldn't jump myself, I'd let the other kids jump for me.

There were moments when I didn't want to live. I didn't know how to live as I was, yet how could a three-year-old say that? I just wanted to go away. Since I couldn't really disappear, I would become the me in the mirror. It probably saved my sanity. If I couldn't do something, I'd just make believe I could, and that I could do it better than anybody else. I got so good at pretending that I practiced and learned all sorts of skills in my head. I taught other kids how to jump rope and play jacks, even though I never physically did those things myself. I practiced hard in my fantasies. I became omnipotent in my fantasies. If I couldn't have power in the "real" world, I could create my own.

Fantasy was my way of protecting myself from the pain of the truth. It hurt when my mother looked at me with pain and grief in her eyes. I could sense that she felt my condition was her fault. I overheard her saying on the phone to a friend that she had asked a priest why this was happening to her child. He told her it was her fault or my father's fault because they must have sinned. I knew it wasn't my fault, but I wished it was. If it had been my fault, maybe she would not have had to blame herself. I felt so often that I had failed her.

Each time a new exercise was presented to her by the doctor-gods, she would try it with me over and over. When I couldn't move my foot or my arm the way they told her to make me, I failed her again.

One day when I was almost four, Aunt Ro invited a few of her friends, my mom and Aunt Kay for coffee. Most of the women had toddlers. While the moms chatted and drank coffee, the kids played wildly in an adjoining room. My mom held me on her lap. She was afraid to leave me alone in the room with the other kids for fear I might get knocked over, hit with a toy or hurt in the roughhousing. My arms weren't strong enough to defend myself, and my back and neck muscles were too weak to maintain a sitting position against much resistance.

One of the women pressed my mom, "Why don't you put her down and let her run around? Don't be so overprotective."

I could feel tears welling up in me. I couldn't tell whether they were my tears, or my mother's. I was sitting on her lap, our bodies pressed together. Her breathing had changed and her muscles had tightened. My mom had assumed that my aunts had told their friends that I had a disability. She was devastated at having to explain about me—the unexplainable. When she told the women that I couldn't walk, it was like she had expelled a dark cloud over the room. I could taste their pity seeping into my cookie, which now had such a bitter taste that it stuck in my throat.

My mother often looked at me sadly. When I was coloring and panting because I was really pressing hard on the crayon, I would look at her and she'd turn away. At those times, I thought she didn't like me, that I made her feel bad because I had to struggle to lift my records or color with my crayons. At the same time she'd push me to do as much for myself as I could, and I often felt pushed beyond my limits. I felt like I was being punished. Day after day, as there was no improvement in my condition, it seemed to me that she felt like she had failed. Occasionally, she turned away from me in shame and despair. It was a sudden turning away; a turning away where her whole body would tense up. Sometimes it would happen when I asked to go to the bathroom or wanted a drink. She'd get gruff with me and I would feel anger in her touch. There were other times when she was gentle with me and very loving, stroking me. Sometimes she was very funny and we would laugh until our eyes filled with tears, and then other times she would grip my body until it hurt, and I would get scared.

It was the worst when my mother withdrew. She would not talk nor look into my eyes, and would move about rigidly, like a robot. The only way I could bring her back was to deliberately cause her to react. I would ask for something she'd assume I really needed to get her to pay attention to me, even though her angry hands scared me. I would work very hard to make her laugh. At the age of four, in order to make my world safe, I knew I had to make my mother happy. I'd think very consciously about what she might like to talk about. I'd remind her of how much fun we had when we went to the park. I was afraid that if she wasn't happy she would leave, either physically or emotionally.

One day, I was trying to get my Betsy-Wetsy's dress off to change her into her nightie for bed. When I pulled too hard, I fell back and to the side on the couch. "Mom!" I called as loudly as I could from that position. I couldn't breathe well with my head tipped back and over. Betsy-Wetsy slid to the floor. "Mom, I fell!"

Mom came in silently. She was tense and had a far-away look in her eyes. She sat me up abruptly, picked up the doll and slammed it into my lap. I winced, smiled up at her, and whispered, "Thanks, Mom. You look pretty." She walked out again without a word.

I looked down at Betsy-Wetsy on my lap. She was naked. I couldn't reach her nightgown and her dress was on the floor. I got a tickle in my throat and started coughing. I coughed quietly. I realized I had to go to the bathroom again.

Mom came in looking angry and tired. "Are you all right?"

"Yes, but I think I have to go to the bathroom."

Something hit me across the face and continued hitting me on my arms and legs. I kept trying to catch my breath. I wanted to run. I wanted to cry, but nothing came out. "Mommy, Mommy," I cried, until I realized it was Mom hitting me.

Time seemed to stand still as the blows kept coming. She

picked me up and carried me to the bathroom, saying, "You're so ungrateful. You don't care about me. I hate you! I hate you! What do you think I am, a slave? You don't appreciate me. You don't deserve anything." She put me on the toilet, directing me to "Go!"

It was very hard to pee. I tried with all my might because I was afraid that if I didn't pee now, she would kill me.

A little pee came out and made noise as it hit the water in the bowl. "That's all? That's what you bothered me for?" Yanking me off the toilet, she pulled up my pants and carried me into the bedroom, pinching my legs and my bottom as she went. She put me down hard into my crib and left, slamming the door behind her.

"Mommy," I sobbed. I was terrified. I would die without her. I cried and choked and gurgled on mucus. I had difficulty swallowing. I cried and shouted for her endlessly, "I'm sorry, I'm sorry." I began to sweat and then felt chilled. Then my bottom started to hurt and my legs and my arms, and I cried in my pain softly to myself. My heart ached for me and for her because I loved her, and I thought she hated me. I prayed to the God in the book Miss Midwood had given me. I prayed that my mother wouldn't go away, while at the same time I was scared of what would happen if she came back into the room.

After a long while, I fell into a fitful sleep. I heard my father come in the front door of the apartment. "Where's Connie?" he asked as he kissed Mom hello.

"She's taking a nap."

Mom came in with a stiff grin, "Your father's home, are you ready for dinner?"

"Yes."

She lifted me up in her arms and suggested that I go to the bathroom before dinner.

We sat down at the table and ate as if nothing had happened. My father told us stories from his work as a plumber. By the end of the meal, my mother was laughing warmly, smiling at me and Dad. I felt good. Mom was happy again. I didn't know how long she would stay happy or when she would get mad at me again. Maybe by the next time, I'd be able to walk and it wouldn't happen. Maybe someone would come and help her so she wouldn't be so tired.

3

CHILDREN WITH
MISSING PARTS

The heat in our apartment was controlled by the landlord. My parents realized that when the apartment was too cold, I got sick; so they were always fighting with the landlord to raise the heat. I was so frightened by the arguing that I would say, "It's okay if I'm cold, I don't mind being cold."

In truth, when I became cold my whole body hurt, and I got weaker. If my arms were cold when I was feeding myself I couldn't feel the spoon. I had to use a lot more energy to feed myself when I was cold, and the more energy I used, the more drained I felt and the colder I became. It takes energy to keep your body warm.

The apartment got colder and colder, and there were more and more fights with the landlord. The next thing I knew, my parents said we were moving to a house of our own.

We moved to Hempstead, Long Island, when I was about four and a half, into a Cape Cod-style house with a front lawn and back yard. There were only three steps to get into the house.

One day I was sitting outside on the lawn in my baby carriage when a little three-year-old girl toddled up to me and asked, "What are you doing in a baby carriage?"

"I can't walk," I replied, and then asked, "What's your name?"

"Susie," she said, "What's yours?"

It startled me. No other kid ever asked me that straight out before; usually they asked about why I was still in a baby carriage, or why I couldn't walk. Anyway, I told her my name, and we became lifelong friends.

I hated to wear shoes that looked forever new, so Susie would wear mine for a while to scuff them up a bit. She would come and knock on my door and ask if I wanted to come out and climb trees. I'd say "Yes." I would be taken outside in my carriage and sit under the tree while Susie climbed. She would describe how things looked and how it felt. I learned how to experience many things through her body.

"Wow, look at this caterpillar! It's all furry on top. Hey, Harold's father's carrying something in a big box. The top of his head is funny. I can't see what's in the box." She squinted and rubbed her eyes. "Ouch! This caterpillar isn't so furry."

Susie was one person who didn't object to my directions. She was my first real friend. If I wanted to dress my doll a certain way and couldn't do it myself, Susie would do it for me. Then she would dress her own doll as she wanted. She was able to remain separate from me and yet loan me her body, using her arms and legs to carry out my will.

I loved the neighborhood kids, except for Tommy. His mother was disabled. She was very cranky and would yell at him and at everyone else. He used to try to pull my hair. I would scream at him and cry for help. Sometimes my mother would come out and yell at him. The other kids seemed to be embarrassed by what he did to me. They usually ignored it when he was mean to me. But once, when he actually did yank my hair, Susie's brother, Richie, came from out of nowhere and knocked him down. Tommy ran away crying.

The other kids in the neighborhood were wonderful. They'd bring games over to play with me, and they'd ask me to go over to their houses. Sometimes I'd be hurt and lonely when they would run off and play in Jeanie's backyard and I couldn't get there. Sometimes they wanted to play baseball and I felt left out, but Susie never let me stay left out. She would ask me to keep score or watch her bat. Summer evenings I could watch the kids play hide-and-seek and Red Rover. They would come up on our porch and talk to me in between games.

Taffy was the first pet I had, a golden cocker spaniel. I got her for Christmas. Three months later, just as she was getting to know me, I had to leave her and go to the hospital.

The hospital had yucky green tile floors and smelled like cleaning fluids. There were many men in white coats and a lot of nurses with white caps. Mommy and Daddy brought me into a room with four cribs. Mommy laid me down in one of them and told me to be a good girl. She kissed me and left. Daddy blew a kiss goodbye and ran after Mommy.

A large black woman in a blue dress took off all my clothes and put a printed elastic-waist skirt and printed elastic-trimmed blouse on me. She was very gentle and kept smiling at me, but I wanted to go home. "Wait until you see what we have for you!"

She lifted me up out of my hospital crib and sat me in this tiny little chair that had wheels.

"What's this?" I asked.

"That's your wheelchair to use while you're here. Let me show you how to work it. Put your hands on the wheels. That's it. Now, push down."

The chair rolled forward. She grabbed the chair in time to prevent me from crashing into a table.

"Hold it!" she exclaimed. "When you want to stop, grab the wheels tight."

I practiced pushing and stopping for a while.

"If you want to go back, grab the wheels and pull up."

I tried it and it worked. This lady was pretty smart.

"Let me show you how to turn. Put one hand down real low on one side and grab the wheel and put your other hand up high on the other side." She put my hands on the wheels and manipulated them as she explained. "Push down with one hand and pull up with the other until your chair turns. Good! Now try it the other way. Turn left, and then turn right." She squatted with her body and pantomimed the motion, and made believe she was in a wheelchair too.

Before the end of the day, I was able to wheel that chair really fast and I loved it. I went around the corner of a hallway all by myself thinking I was hiding from everyone. The only thing was that I didn't have enough hand strength to lock and unlock my brakes.

I didn't know what the hospital people wanted. I guess they were testing to see why I wasn't working properly— why I wasn't able to walk, and why I wasn't getting stronger. They tested for muscle problems, nerve problems, brain problems, hormone problems and any other problems they could think of. The tests felt like torture. They gave me an EMG where they stuck needles into my muscles, sent electricity into them and read what electric impulses the muscles produced on their own. The pain was so bad that I thought they were trying to kill me. I knew this place must be where they made the screaming war and horror movies that my mommy wouldn't let me watch. I thought, "I'm not supposed to be here."

I didn't like to wear the hospital printed skirts with elastic in the waist and the little puffed-sleeve blouses with elastic. I wanted my own clothes. I didn't like to have to scream for the nurse ten or fifteen times in the night when my leg hurt and I needed to be turned. I hated the place: the smells, the colors, the food, the sounds. It was filled with people who were deformed and wore strange things, and children with missing parts. I wasn't like them. I knew I could walk, the Connie in the mirror said so.

"Come on, Connie, you have PT now," barked a woman

in blue as she wheeled me too quickly down the hall. She wheeled me into a big room with cots and mats and all kinds of big metal equipment. There were big people and little people half undressed with their arms or legs being moved in weird positions by machines or people in white. It smelled like sweat.

"So! You're here for some physical therapy, eh?" asked a man in white, stooping over to stare at my face.

"I don't know," I blinked.

"Take her over here."

The woman in blue parked me near a bench, locked my brakes, and left me there. Pretty soon, another woman, who spoke a little like my grandmother, asked me to get on the bench.

"I can't. I can't walk."

"Sure you can," she smiled. "We're going to show you." She lifted me onto the bench and sat me on the edge. She let go. I started to fall. She caught me. "Sit up now. Come on, you can do it."

For the next ten minutes I exhausted myself out of fear of falling, and fear of this woman getting mad at me and leaving me there, or hitting me.

Finally the man in white came over. "Maria, she can't sit up. Lay her down and see what you can do with those legs."

Maria laid me down, took my skirt off and my shoes and socks. She lifted up my leg. "Hold it up now. Tight as you can."

She let go of my leg and it fell hard onto the bench. She tried again. "No, no, no. Hold your leg up."

"I can't," I cried. "I can't walk!"

"Yes, you can. You can walk if you want to. You just don't want to. Hold your leg up!"

My leg dropped again. The man came over and they mumbled something about flaccid and other big words that I knew meant trouble for me.

"Test her arms, Maria."

Maria bent my arm. "Push against my hand, hard."
I struggled and her arm didn't move. "I can't."
"Yes, you can."
"No, I can't."
"Why?" asked Maria.
I thought for a few moments. I was confused. They were telling me I could walk, but I knew I couldn't. Sometimes I thought I could because I looked like I could, and I wanted to.
"Because I don't want to. I'm tired."
"You're lazy," retorted Maria. "I have a little boy younger than you and he runs around and climbs stairs. He's tough. Pick up your leg. Come on, kick me." She put my foot against her stomach.
"Nooooo!" I screamed and burst into body-wrenching tears of frustration and confusion.
The black woman in blue who had shown me how to use the wheelchair appeared from nowhere. She picked me up and put me back in the wheelchair, telling me, "Don't be a cry-baby. You're fine." She smiled at me and wheeled me back down the hall to my room to wait for dinner.
I had to stay in the hospital in New York City for five weeks. I was allowed to come home on weekends, and my mother was only allowed to visit me every Tuesday for two hours. I thought, "They finally caught up with me. I'll have to stay here until I agree to walk, or I will never go home." While they did bring me home on the weekend, they always took me back to the hospital. I would get stomach cramps as we drove through the Midtown Tunnel back into the city.

Suppertime was a particularly hard time for me at the hospital. I missed my parents, my mom's food, my dad's stories, and I hated being surrounded by people with strange contraptions who were dribbling their food and talking in languages I didn't understand with contorted faces. I always cried through dinner. After dinner, at story-time, I would sob silently with my head down, too defeated and too tired to cry aloud anymore. One night Dr. Deaver, the head of the hospital, came on the ward. He knelt down beside me and said, "What have we here?"

Speechless in my sorrow, I couldn't answer him. All I could do was stare back at him, my eyes brimming with tears.

"What's the matter?"

All I could muster was another look.

"Do you miss your mommy and daddy?"

I nodded.

"Come with me," and he picked me up in his arms, took me to his big office, sat me on his desk and called my parents.

"Hello? Mr. and Mrs. Panzarino? This is Dr. Deaver at the Institute of Rehabilitation Medicine. Connie is here and she misses you very much and would like to talk to you."

He handed the receiver to me. I held it with two hands. "Mommy?!" I said and started sobbing, "I want to come home." My mother started crying too, and my dad began comforting her. Meanwhile, Taffy jumped up on the table and ate my dad's dinner. I heard him yelling at the dog. I was laughing and crying. Dr. Deaver looked very confused.

The children with missing parts really scared me. I didn't know if they were going to take my parts off, nor did I understand how those kids lost their parts. Did they lose them because somebody screwed up with a test and they fell off? Did they not do their exercises and the therapists took off those parts as punishment? Or were their mothers angry with them, the way my mother got angry with me, and then took pieces off them? I heard that some of them were born that way and I thought, "God, they must have a worse time of it than I do." So I felt sorry for them as well. But mostly it scared me because I didn't know what had happened to the pieces that were missing.

I met one young teenager who couldn't pee by herself, and I wondered how they broke her pee thing. Then I found out that she'd been shot, accidently. The world out there became even more scary. I thought that only my mommy got angry and that only landlords were mean. Suddenly, it felt like there was a connection between all that anger and being in the hospital, and I didn't know what to make of it. I only knew I was trapped there.

I was sitting in my hospital room, looking out the window at the Empire State Building. It was a Wednesday. Mommy had come yesterday to see me and I was thinking about her. All of a sudden Dr. Deaver walked into the room. "Here she is."

"Mommy! Daddy!" I shouted.

Mommy hugged and kissed me and so did Daddy. "We're taking you home, honey." Mommy dressed me in my own clothes from home while the doctor talked to them.

"Basically, according to the tests, she appears to have a neuromuscular disease which affects voluntary muscles. She has amyotonia congenita."

"But there's no treatment?" asked my dad.

"None per se. With amyotonias, well, we just try to manage their care with therapy and braces to keep them from curving and to keep them from getting stiff. There are some experimental treatments we may want to try at some point if, of course, you're willing."

Now I had a disease. It didn't seem like I had a disease. It seemed like they were saying I *was* a disease. I knew I was different. Now I had a name for the difference, like being Italian or Jewish. I was an Amyotonia. I didn't understand if that meant that I would never walk, or if all it meant was lack of muscle tone. I didn't know that most children with this disease die before they're five years old. No one said anything to me about that.

Mommy picked me up and carried me toward the door. "Wait!" I screamed. "My chair!"

"No, honey, that chair belongs to the hospital. You have to leave it here."

All of a sudden there was a big pain inside my chest. I thought of how awful it would be to go home and sit immobile forever in my little chair at the table. I wanted a chair with wheels. I was being torn in two. It was as though part of me was staying there and the other part of me was going home to be trapped again. I hung my head over Mom's shoulder. Maybe I had to leave the chair behind as punishment for not learning to walk while I was there.

After five weeks of insane tests and evaluations I returned home for good. I had failed. I still couldn't walk. I was glad I had failed. It felt like getting even for being sent there in the first place. But I also felt guilty for failing.

We got a television. Mom and I had lots of fun with it. It was good to get home to my puppy. When I had seen her on weekend visits home, she often forgot who I was and snapped at me. She was a very nervous pup. I'd get mad at her because she wouldn't come to me when I called, and I couldn't run after her. I didn't think she cared about me very much, but I liked her.

I was given experimental hormone pills which were hard to swallow. I choked on them a lot, so I tried to avoid taking them. I didn't know then that the hormones themselves might also be dangerous to me. Sometimes, I saved them in my hand. Then, while I was sitting on the toilet, I'd throw the orange ones into the slots in the bathroom radiator. The big red pills wouldn't fit in the slots, so I tried to press them between my legs into the toilet. This didn't work very well, because my mother saw them in the toilet and told the doctor that they weren't dissolving in my stomach. So, I decided to give the red ones to Taffy. The next year Taffy died of cancer. She went to the vet one day and never came back. I always thought that she got cancer from the pills. I felt guilty, but glad to be alive. She sacrificed her life for me. Luckily, by then the doctor stopped prescribing the pills anyway.

4

HARD FLOORS

Before my stay in the hospital, my life had consisted of getting up in the morning after my father went to work, having breakfast with my mother and playing most of the day while she worked. Sometimes she would take me to the store. Once in a while a neighbor would come in for coffee and bring their child along for me to play with, or I would sit outside in the afternoon and play with the kids in the neighborhood.

Suddenly there was a new regimen. I had to wear painful metal braces with leather straps on my legs, and a tight corset so my back would stay straight. I had to stand in my braces without moving for two hours each day, an hour in the morning and an hour in the afternoon.

My mother would brush my hair while I was standing in my braces. It was very long—well below my waist. I mostly wore my hair in braids, but sometimes it hung loose down my back. It would often be snarled. It hurt to brush it out, but my mother gave me a lot of attention in the loving way she took care of my dark, wavy Italian hair. Sometimes on hot summer days she would put it in an upsweep of curls piled on top of my head. My hair was pretty, and it wasn't disabled. Mom loved my hair. But one day she cut it and saved my braids. She said that having the long hair was a lot more trouble for her to wash, and it got dirty easier because it would get into everything. I couldn't help thinking that she cut it off because I couldn't walk.

Since my knees and ankles didn't go straight the way other people's did, my mother had to lay me down on the table and stretch them twice a day. It was painful. Standing on the braces also stretched my hips and knees, which added to the pain. She also had to do leg and arm exercises with me several times a day.

"Mom," I said, wiping my mouth after my last bite of the fresh peach I had eaten for dessert, "can I watch TV?"

"No, you have to do your new exercise. Frank, take her in and put her on the floor."

My father carried me into the living room, and laid me on the living room floor. "Now you roll over and over until you reach the other side of the room, and then you roll all the way back. When you're all done with your exercise you can watch TV."

"But I can't," I wailed, thinking to myself that I couldn't even turn over in bed.

"You try!" came a retort from the kitchen, followed by a clatter of dishes in the sink.

"Here, I'll help you get started." Dad lifted my arm up alongside my head and crossed my leg over so that I was beginning to tilt on my side. He rocked me back and forth saying encouragingly, "See, you can do it!" He brushed the hair gently out of my eyes, "Now, just push yourself over and keep going." He walked out of the room, leaving me on my side.

I rocked and pushed and panted. I finally got myself pushed over so that I was on my stomach. My nose and chin smacked hard against the wood floor. "Mom," I cried out. "Mommy, help me. Please? I can't do it. It hurts." I began sobbing and pushing hard with my hand and leg to tilt myself back away from the floor. I couldn't push myself back enough to roll over onto my back, but each time I pushed, it alleviated the pain in my face for the few seconds I could hold myself. "Mom," I cried.

"Come on, you can do it. Don't be such a baby." Mom pushed just enough for me to gain the momentum to flip over onto my back. I tried to catch her eye as she stood there, but she wouldn't look at me. She left the room and went back to cleaning the kitchen.

I heard a knock at the back door. "No, Susie, I'm sorry but Connie has to do exercises after dinner and she can't come out to play until she's finished." My stomach began to hurt. I didn't know why she was tormenting me, but then I did know; I had failed. Again, I thought, this was my punishment for failing to walk.

"See, there you go. Look how far you've rolled since I put you down on the floor." Dad came walking heavily into the room. "Now, put your arm up like this, and your leg over like that, and just keep rolling," He put my arm up and my leg over and left the room again.

I knew I could get forward onto my face again if I tried really hard, but I also knew it would hurt. "Mommy, Daddy, Mommy, Daddy, I can't do this. I have to get up now!" I felt like biting my arms. I hated my parents, the hard floor and my body that didn't work right. I was exhausted. I decided to make believe that I had been thrown into a dungeon by a wicked witch. I fell asleep on my side.

When I woke up, the leg and arm that were against the floor were burning with pain. I screamed and cried out loud.

"All right, all right, that's enough of this," Mom snapped. She picked me up off the floor and put me over her shoulder. I winced from the blood rushing back into my arms and legs and because I half expected her to hit me. She sat me on the couch. "You sit here and play with your toys. I'll put you to bed as soon as I finish the sink. We'll try again tomorrow." She kissed me and went into the kitchen.

• • •

Sometimes I imagined that I would get up and walk and show them all. But then I thought they might beat me because they would know that all this time I had been lying. I wasn't really lying, but I didn't know that. When I couldn't do the exercises, my father said I was lazy and my mother lost patience and hit me. I didn't know that the doctors had told my mother that if she did everything they told her to do, I would be walking by the time I was ten years old. Since I wasn't improving, Mom thought that either she or I wasn't doing enough. She began to handle me roughly and hurt me when she took care of me on the toilet. I cried more than I thought any child should ever have to cry. Mom cried too. I was five, and she was twenty-five.

Since standing in my braces was such an awful experience, my mother would often put me by the front door to look out. I would hold onto the door knob for support. My mother would stand behind me so I wouldn't fall. I would watch the cars going by and wave to the neighbors, and soon I'd forget about the pain.

One day she went to answer the phone and I forgot she wasn't behind me. I was rocking back and forth and playing with the knob, and getting lost in the leaves swirling to the ground. All of a sudden I lost my balance and fell over backwards like a tree. My head throbbed from hitting the floor. My mother came running in and scooped me up. I had realized the power of single-handedly throwing myself to the floor. If I couldn't stand up alone, at least I could fall down alone.

When I was six years old I finally got my own wheelchair. It wasn't a tiny little wheelchair like the one I had used in the hospital. It was bigger, because I was supposed to wear my braces all the time. The braces took up room, so the doctors prescribed a big wheelchair. But it was so big, I couldn't wheel it.

My parents told me that I had to push the awful chair around the house, even though it was too big for me to maneuver. I could not do it. I could wheel it only about half an inch a minute. I would jab my thumb nail into the wheel, push with all my might, and rock my body so the chair would move a little bit. It felt like someone's idea of a bad joke. But at least I was out of the baby carriage, and the new chair was high enough that I was actually able to reach tables.

When spring came I could finally sit outside again. One day when the trees were beginning to bloom, I sat waiting for Susie to come out. Maybe she would come over and play with me. I hadn't seen much of her lately because she and the other kids were into roller-skating. Perhaps Susie felt like playing a sitting-down game for a change. The day was too beautiful to spend alone. It was hard being so immobile on such a great day, but I wouldn't mind if I had someone to talk to.

Just then Susie came out of her house. I yelled, "Hi, Sue. Want to come over?" To my dismay, she held up those shiny steel roller skates and shouted, "I'm going to skate, Conn, but I'll come over there and talk to you while I put them on."

My eyes filled with tears. I blinked them back as Susie approached and resolved to look at the skates. Maybe the skates wouldn't be so hard to look at if I smiled and pretended to take an interest in them.

Susie strolled up to me and sat down in a clatter as the steel of the skates hit the cement driveway. "They're new," she said with a grin. "Want to try them on?"

She startled me. I didn't know quite what to say, but I was determined to take an interest. "Yeah, okay."

We put them on, laughing. A few kids gathered around and stared. Susie placed my feet, skates and all, on the ground and began pushing my wheelchair up and down the front walk. "Hang on, Conn. Tell me if I'm going too fast now."

The other kids began skating along side and behind me. They began shouting. "Hey! Wait for me!"

"Not so fast!"

"I'll race you."

"Keep out of my way." I shouted back. I was moving with the kids, more a part of them, a part of a whole. The kids had always sought me out on rainy days when they couldn't go out and run or when they were recovering from the measles and had to stay quiet. At those times we were bosom buddies—allies on the immobile front. But when the sun shone and everyone was healthy, I was often abandoned.

After about ten minutes of skating, I said, "I'm bushed, gang. I'm going to sit down for a while. You go ahead and skate, Susie."

A week later my friend Lucille got a jump rope and I was "steady-ender" for the rest of the year. I learned to play all kinds of games with my new wheelchair. Even though I couldn't wheel it myself, it still gave me more mobility than the baby carriage. I used to play "train" with Susie. She'd sit on my footrests, I'd bend over her, and she'd pull us along with her feet while both of us yelled "choo-choo!" This game was fun until one day I bent over a little too far and fell head over heels over Susie and onto the floor. We both cracked up laughing. I didn't get hurt, but boy did we scare my mother.

Somehow my family survived. My father started his own plumbing business. My mother was his secretary at night, his wife, the homemaker, my nurse, my physical therapist, the cook, the laundress, the chauffeur, the gardener, the message taker and on and on. I wondered at her. I worried about her. I loved her, and I hated her for not giving up. The way she had to live made me feel guilty.

Occasionally she could not bear up. She would threaten to leave me somewhere. When my physical demands were more than she could tolerate, the abuse cycle would begin again. I was caught between compassion for her, fear of her anger, and fear of abandonment. When I was bad, or my parents were overwhelmed, they said things like, "We could just put you in a home." I thought they didn't really want me, because I was such a big burden.

Mom needed to do the shopping, but she couldn't afford a babysitter. She had to take me with her, and leave me in the car for the hour it took to shop. She would peek out at me through the store window to see if I was okay. I was so low in the seat that I couldn't really see her. Sometimes I would get cold, especially in winter. I thought I would freeze to death before she came back. I panicked when there was a big bug crawling over my leg or crawling across the roof of the car towards me. I feared that Mommy might never come back. Sometimes I fantasized that somebody else might find me. An hour seemed like such a long time to sit alone in the car. If I was crying when she came back, she would hit me.

It always seemed like I belonged to my mother. Since she took total care of me, she had total power over me. She told me what to do, what to wear, what she thought of what I did. I believed I had to please her—not that I didn't want to. I liked to please her, but I thought I *had* to please her because my life depended on her.

Sometimes I thought Mom seemed angry when other people were affectionate with me. She gave my grandmother dirty looks when she was caressing me or cuddling me. My mother would say "You're going to spoil her" or "What are you doing that for?" I thought maybe I didn't deserve the affection. She did the same thing when my father hugged me. It was as if she was the only one allowed to hug me. Maybe she thought I didn't want to be hugged. I was told to kiss people hello, but sometimes when they hugged or kissed me on their own, Mom didn't seem to like it. It was all very confusing.

Mom and I spent a lot of special time together. I could talk to her about things I couldn't talk about with anyone else. I could ask her if my Ginny doll minded that I couldn't braid her hair by myself. Mom was the one that consoled me when other kids ran off to play without me or when I spilled food on myself while eating. Sometimes she had no patience for me. Other times Mom seemed a pillar of strength. At those times I could lean on her and depend on her for comfort. She interpreted the world to me and helped me learn that I had a place in this world, even if I was different.

Sometimes when we sat alone on the couch at home or on a bench in the park, she would tell me how she felt about her sisters or something my father's mother said. I knew it was adult business and I wasn't expected to understand. She just needed me to listen. Other times, Mom would very intensely explain things that left me feeling bewildered. Like one morning when I was six, when she picked me up out of my bed and carried me into her room.

"Daddy went to work, so you can lay on his side of the bed," Mommy said tucking me in the bed next to her. "You be Daddy."

She climbed in beside me and we went back to sleep as we did other mornings. When I woke up, we started talking about what I wanted for breakfast and what I might do that day.

"Do you know where babies come from?" Mom asked me.

"No. Are we going to get one?"

"No, but let me tell you about where babies come from. Girls have eggs inside of them, and every month an egg comes down from one side or the other, and if God wants you to get pregnant and have a baby, he makes the egg turn into a baby. If he doesn't want you to have a baby, the egg breaks open and blood comes out a special little hole that girls have. It's the same hole that babies come out of. God never wants you to have a baby if you're not married, though."

I lay there, wondering if God would ever want me to have a baby. I wasn't sure why Mom was telling me this. I thought maybe I should pray or something.

It seemed like I was so totally a part of her that when she wasn't the one caretaking me, I didn't exist to her. If I was in a room with my father reading a book while he read the newspaper, he might smile at me once in a while. I would catch his eye as I was turning pages, or he might pat my head as he walked by me on the way back from the bathroom. We would be together, yet separate in the same room. But when my mother was in the room with me, I felt acutely aware of her presence. Her eyes were always on me. Her mothering "antennae" were so intensely tuned to my needs that I think she often didn't know where her wants began and mine left off. Sometimes she would get up and reposition me because I looked uncomfortable to her. Most of the time she was right, but sometimes she was wrong. If she was thirsty or hungry, she would assume I must be too. When I was thirsty, and she wasn't, she would often tell me I didn't need a drink. She would say "I'm cold" and get up and put my sweater on me. It was hard to know if I could ever exist separate from her, so I couldn't seem to relax and be with her the way I could with my father or my other relatives. It was hard to know who I was, how to be myself and be with other people, and how much of me was her.

I got sick a lot and it made things very hard. Being sick meant more doctor's bills, more stress on my family, more guilt and more anger. A simple cold could keep me in bed for weeks. My grandmother often came from Brooklyn when I was sick and stayed with us until I got well.

But most of the time, Grandma wasn't there and Mom had a lot to do. Often I had to be left alone in the house while Mom went to empty the garbage. If she started talking to a neighbor, or stopped to check out the flowers, my heart would pound because I would think that since she didn't seem to want to come back, maybe she really wouldn't. It was hard to know when I was safe.

One day Mommy went out of the house to empty the garbage. I became afraid because I was alone and began rocking to a fantasy of riding a bouncing tree branch to escape my fear. When I came to my senses, I realized she hadn't come in yet, and the room was filled with smoke. She had gotten involved with talking to a neighbor. I saw the kitchen turn bright orange. I screamed, "Mommy, Mommy!"

She yelled, "Wait a minute, I'll be right there. You're okay."

I started yelling, "Fire! Fire! Fire!"

Susie's father heard me and ran into the kitchen with my mother at his heels. "Cover the frying pan!" my mother shouted. I heard pot lids clanking and steam hissing. I couldn't quite see what was happening. They opened the kitchen door to let the smoke out. The kitchen slowly returned to its natural pink. My mother looked at me and laughed sarcastically, saying, "I never know when to believe you."

When I was seven, my parents sent me to catechism to prepare for my first holy communion. My teacher was a wonderful person who was always smiling. All the nuns seemed to really love each other. I would see them walking arm-in-arm and embracing each other when they met or parted.

In catechism, I got to meet and learn with a large group of children. We were taught songs, prayers and stories about how good Jesus was. I learned about all the miracles he performed and the people like me that he cured. I had a lot of private talks with Jesus, and his mother Mary, about cures. I didn't really need a cure, since I still thought I was not walking on purpose. But sometimes I prayed that Jesus would make me walk in spite of myself.

The last day before my first communion, Sister Mary kissed me on the cheek, saying, "You're such a good girl. You answered all the questions correctly, and now you're ready to receive Jesus."

Tears welled up in my eyes. How could she say I was good when I still couldn't walk and I made my mommy so miserable. I suddenly knew that I wanted to be just like Sister Mary. "When I grow up, can I become a nun like you?"

"No, darling. I'm afraid that to be a nun and to serve God you have to be able to walk and take care of yourself. But that is a sweet thought."

Even God was rejecting me. I got very quiet.

5

PARTY HATS
AND BASKETS

"Connie, how would you like to go to school?" Mom asked.

My mind raced. Every day I watched the kids in the neighborhood coming home from school, shouting and dancing and jumping in the streets. "Yes!" I shouted.

My parents took me in to see the classroom. My eyes danced around the room. I'd be able to sit at the tables with the other children and do things with them. While my mother and father met with the principal and the nurse, the teacher let me stay in the classroom. They served milk and cookies. I was beaming. All these kids were my size and none of them had missing parts.

Mommy came back about half an hour later and picked me up off the seat. She hugged me gently and sorrowfully. My dad put his arm around her. As we walked down the hall and out the door of the school, Mrs. Piper, the nurse, said, "I'm sorry, but I just can't take the responsibility of lifting her on and off the toilet. We'll have a teacher get in touch with you soon to set something up."

I wondered if she was saying that I could never go to the bathroom in school.

As we got into the car, Dad said, puzzled, "What a shame. That school even has a ramp for the wheelchair. They could put her class on the first floor."

"Well, Frank, she is getting heavy, you know," Mom replied, "and she's going to grow."

"Am I going to school tomorrow?" I asked eagerly.

"No," they said in unison.

"You're going to have a teacher come to the house to teach you because the nurse can't lift you onto the toilet if you have to go to the bathroom," Mom explained.

I hated the school, the nurse, the kids, my parents, and my fat body that had to pee even when I didn't want it to.

My first teacher's name was Mrs. Friefeld. She came from three-thirty to four-thirty every day. She gave me five to six hours of homework to do the following day until she came. I was bright, so I learned to read, write and do math pretty early. She also gave me some creative projects, like writing about things in the encyclopedia, drawing pictures of birds, making reports or writing poems. But when she came, Susie and all the other children on the block were just arriving home from school. My schooltime was their playtime, and my playtime was their schooltime.

In third grade, I had a different teacher, who came earlier in the day. I got to see the neighborhood kids more, but because they all had different homework, and had new friends they met in school that I didn't know, it was hard to talk to them. They wanted to talk about things that happened during the day. It made me lonely. When they talked about how they hated school, I thought they were crazy. But then I began to hate school too because it took the kids away from me.

In fourth grade, I had a teacher named Mrs. Summers, who thought that since I was disabled anyway, I shouldn't have to suffer through learning anything. She taught me how to make party hats and baskets. They weren't even real baskets, they were paper. I tried putting things into them and they ripped. I got so bored I would rock and rub my thighs together. She didn't even notice. She was so busy cutting and folding and getting excited about the paper things she was making to hang in my window that I didn't even have to be there.

I almost didn't pass fourth grade, because she hadn't taught me anything. My parents began to realize that they were not seeing tests or compositions I was writing. They called the school to complain. The school sent Mrs. Friefeld back for the last six weeks of the school year. She was tough and in the remaining time taught me everything I needed to know to pass fourth grade.

For the next two years, I had a nice, quiet, gentle man who came from one to two o'clock every day. Mr. Jacob was his name. He used to go to different disabled kids at different times during the day. He didn't give me much homework, and when he did, I did it in twenty minutes. It was easy and I could still see Susie after school each day.

Twice a year, I went to the hospital in New York City for checkups. As we drove through the Midtown Tunnel one January, I began to get stomach cramps. "Mommy," I moaned, "I have a stomach ache."

"We're only five minutes from the hospital," she replied. "She always gets a stomach ache when we come here," she whispered to my father.

"She eats too much," he retorted.

Masturbating didn't work for getting rid of diarrhea cramps the way it did when I had to pee. There was nothing I could do but wait and hope that my parents wouldn't get mad at me and leave me at the hospital to punish me.

We pulled up in the circular drive at the hospital entrance. Dad got the wheelchair out of the trunk, while Mom strained to lift me out of the car.

"Why don't you go park the car while I take her to the bathroom?"

"Okay, Annie," replied Dad cheerily.

Mom struggled to put me on the toilet in the small booth. It was getting more and more difficult for her to balance me over her shoulder while she pulled my pants up after I went. Panting, she put me back into the chair. "Wait here while I go to the bathroom."

I could see myself in the mirror. My hair and clothes were messed up, and I looked fat. I was probably smaller than other children my age, but too big to be carried around. I was put on a lot of diets. Some of them were supposed to help me walk, others were to help me lose weight. My cousin Vinny was fatter than me and he didn't have to go on diets. I had to drink skim milk, and was not allowed to eat ice cream or sugary stuff. I was told that other kids run around so they burn off the sugar, but since I didn't run around and exercise the way the doctors wanted me to, I shouldn't have sweets because they made me fat. Family friends often brought me presents because of my disability, and the most common present was candy. My mother would take it away and ration it out. When I was sick, they let me eat the candy.

"Ready?" Mom pushed me in my wheelchair out the bathroom door. We met Dad in the lobby and went up to the children's unit. Dad was carrying my braces. We waited for hours in the hall with a lot of other parents, children and screaming babies. There were not enough seats, so parents took turns sitting down, offering seats to one another. Lots of people in white coats passed us by. One of them walked with crutches. I wondered if she was a doctor. Another woman in white came out of the physical therapy room and waved us in.

We went into a little booth with a curtain around it. "Please undress her and put her up on the table." The woman disappeared in a swish of curtains.

Dad lifted me up onto the table and Mom undressed me silently. She put my clothes on the wheelchair. I laid there naked, getting goosebumps. Dad propped my braces up on the wheelchair and cleared his throat. He looked at the floor, nervous or embarrassed, I couldn't tell which.

After a long time, the curtains swished wide open and a crowd of doctors appeared. The head doctor smiled at me and nodded at my parents. He then lectured to the doctors for fifteen minutes in language I could not understand while he pointed to various parts of my body and flopped my arms and legs around. "Stick out your tongue, darling. See! See! Take a look."

One by one the doctors peered around him at my tongue, nodding. I felt sick to my stomach.

"Where are her braces? Are those her braces? Let me see them," the head doctor demanded. "How old is she now?"

"Eight," I said proudly.

He looked at my mother.

"Eight," she nodded.

"Eight," he said, nodding and smiling at me. "She's doing great. A little too fat, but otherwise she's doing great. It's so hard with these children. The only enjoyment they have is eating."

I wondered what he would do if he knew how good it felt to rub my legs together.

The doctor started to say goodbye and leave. My father grabbed him by the arm and whispered. "What about . . . other children . . . will they . . . handicapped . . . normal . . . Are there tests . . . ? Should we . . . ?"

My mother had stopped dressing me. Her full attention was on the doctor's face.

"There's no problem. The chances of this kind of thing," he waved toward me, "happening again is so small. I would go ahead."

I saw my parents breathe a sigh of relief and smile at each other shyly.

In April of that year, Mom became pregnant. My mother was not really supposed to lift me while she was pregnant. This meant that if I had to use the bathroom I had to wait either for a neighbor or my father. We had some horrendous battles ending in tears and urine on the floor. Then Mom would lift me anyway. Once she looked at me screaming, "If this child is born without arms and legs it will be your fault because you couldn't wait to go to the bathroom."

That December, my brother was born. Luckily he was normal. He was named Frank after my father. My father hung a sign outside the house that read, "It's a boy!" He was very excited. We hugged each other.

Soon the baby's needs were competing with my own. Neither of us could dress ourselves or go to the bathroom independently. He was a colicky baby, who needed a lot of attention. I feared that my already overtaxed mother would disintegrate under the extra burden, but she didn't. In fact, she seemed pleased. She never left my brother alone in the house, so I felt safer. He was a kind of insurance which guaranteed that she wouldn't leave.

I wasn't sure how I could really be a big sister since I had so little mobility. Mom found ways for me to help, though, like singing or talking to Frankie, listening for him if she went downstairs to put wash in, and even helping to feed him.

My brother was somewhat hyperactive. Maybe it was just that my mother wasn't used to having a kid that could run around, but he was really quick on his feet. He talked baby talk. My parents thought it was cute, since I had never gone through a baby talk stage.

. . .

I had a corner desk in my room. At the time I wanted to be a scientist, so I had bacteria growing in petri dishes on my desk. When he was eighteen months old, Frankie liked to chin up on the desk and pull the whole thing over. The little germs would fly all over my room. I thought I would be poisoned. I kept my door shut. Then one day he was tall enough to reach the doorknob. The little monster was actually growing! I gave up growing bacteria or leaving anything vulnerable out.

Frankie also did things that were considered normal for siblings, except that I couldn't fight back. He hit me, and got into the habit of biting me. My mother didn't want to be afraid to leave me alone in the room with him, so one day she bit him back to teach him what it felt like. It worked. He never bit me again.

As he got older, he learned to be really helpful. He learned to work my foot pedals, lift my feet on or off the pedals, or wheel my chair. He became my arms and legs at times. Once, under my direction, he opened up all the walnuts on the coffee table in the livingroom. After we ate the nutmeat, we glued the empty walnut shells together and put them back in the bowl. At Sunday dinner my grandfather kept opening the walnuts saying, "What the hell is going on? Where'd you get these walnuts? They're no good!" We laughed so hard I started to choke, and Frankie nearly wet his pants.

The summer that I was nine, my parents sent me to day camp. It was held at the United Cerebral Palsy Center. The ratio of volunteers to disabled children was one-to-one. Each camper had a volunteer for the day, which for me meant that I could run here and there in my wheelchair because I had someone to push me. I became so active and involved in camp activities that I was assigned one volunteer in the morning and another one in the afternoon. Otherwise I would wear them out.

Lois was a volunteer I met at camp. She would also baby-sit me on Saturday nights at home. Lois was beautiful. I'd stay up as late as I could, playing games and talking to her. I was torn between going to sleep so that she would give me a hug and kiss goodnight, or trying to stay awake to be with her. Then Lois began to bring her boyfriend to babysit with her. I hated that. He was nice, but I wanted Lois all to myself.

The volunteers were great. They cheered us on to win contests, make beautiful things in arts and crafts, and pick flowers when we weren't supposed to. They would never help us do anything dangerous, but they let us be "bad" and learn the consequences in a reasonable way.

One day, as we were making model cars for a race, I directed my volunteer, "Give me Billy's car."

She did.

"Hey!" Billy yelled at her. "That's my car."

"Connie told me to take your car, so I had to," said my volunteer.

"Give me my car back!" Billy directed his volunteer. "Connie, don't you take my car again without asking."

And so I learned to ask first, if I wanted something. This was different than having to ask for help with my physical needs. Camp was great. I never had to wait to go to the bathroom or have a drink of water, and I learned to paint, shoot a rifle, play baseball and swim.

Swimming was wonderful. In the water, I was light and buoyant. I could move! But I was also scared, because I was afraid I would drown. Sometimes the water was so cold it made me weak and shivery, and it gave me a headache. My neck muscles were weak, so my face sometimes slipped under water, and I couldn't breathe. But I liked swimming because I could stand up in the water. With a tube around me to hold me up, I could actually walk around the pool.

I also learned to make friends with other children with disabilities. We had a kinship and yet were different. I still thought I could really walk. Besides, I looked more normal than the children with cerebral palsy. The children with muscular dystrophy were still mostly able to walk, but I knew they were going to get worse and die. I didn't know anyone else with amyotonia. Every summer and at every special Christmas party, I looked for someone like me.

When I was ten, my mother became pregnant again. Since I was bigger than I had been when she was pregnant with my brother, it was even more dangerous for her to lift me. She could not help me go to the bathroom. Sometimes my Uncle Pete, my father's brother, came to lift me, and once in a while a neighbor would help. Mostly, I limited my fluid intake and waited for Dad to come home.

When my sister, Patricia, was born, I was really glad because Mom had a girl. When she came home from the hospital, my mother nursed her. She looked like a little pigeon with her mouth open wanting to eat, so we nicknamed her "Pidgie."

The next night, a group of relatives came to see the baby. I began having this strange pain in my stomach. I thought my pants were too tight. My mother loosened my pants, but it didn't help. My grandmother took me to the toilet because my mother wasn't supposed to lift me yet. It still didn't help. I couldn't get comfortable, and the pain gnawed at me most of the night. The next morning the doctor came. He said I had appendicitis. That afternoon I went to the hospital to have my appendix removed.

When I got back home, life seemed really hard and confusing. Mom seemed more worn out than ever. Although Pidgie was not colicky, slept well and was a very beautiful baby, Frankie was very active and I still needed a lot of care.

When Pidgie was about seven months old, my mother and I both noticed that she wasn't sitting up as well as my brother had, and couldn't reach out for things without falling. Mom and I looked at each other fearfully as we watched her struggle. I think we both knew that Pidgie had what I had. When she was ten or eleven months old, my parents took her to see Dr. Millerat, the head of the Institute for Muscle Diseases in New York City.

Dr. Millerat had had a larynx operation because he had cancer, so he had to speak through his esophagus, which made his voice sound deep and gravelly. While he was discussing my sister's diagnosis, she sat on my mother's lap mimicking him. My mother was torn between being devastated that Pidgie also had amyotonia, being validated because she had been right, and being embarrassed because her baby was sitting there mumbling, "Mrs. Panzarino, we regret to inform you . . . congenital, like . . . recessive genes . . . several generations back, perhaps . . . no way of knowing" in a deep-throated stomach voice. Pidgie, like me, talked fluently and clearly at this age.

A few months later, they put Pidgie through an electromylogram test. Frankie and I went with them because there was no one to take care of us. My sister screamed for what seemed like an eternity. My mother was upset in the hallway, holding my little brother, who, at three, looked terrified. I became sick to my stomach with memories of my own EMG.

It was difficult for my mother to give us the care my sister and I needed, raise my brother, and be a wife to my father. Often my needs weren't met, or I had to wait a very long time. Sometimes Pidgie's needs weren't met either.

"Mom, I have to go to the bathroom," Pidgie sang out.

"Damn," I thought to myself, "so do I."

"Just a minute," Mom replied.

"Pidgie, you can't have to go again. You just went two hours ago," I snapped. "*I* have to go to the bathroom. I haven't gone since this morning."

"Yeah, but I have a cold," she whined. "Mommy said I have to drink a lot of juice and that means I have to go a lot."

"Yeah, it's always something with you. You always need something."

"Shut up!" Pidgie blew at me hard.

"Keep your damn germs to yourself!" I cried. I blew back at her. "Mom, Pidgie is blowing her germs at me."

Mom appeared from nowhere and smacked Pidgie across the face. "You stop that, Missy. It's bad enough having one of you sick." She unlocked Pidgie's brakes and wheeled her off to the bedroom to put her on the bedpan. I heard more slapping and shouting from the other room. I heard Pidgie crying. My stomach hurt.

"How am I going to get to go to the bathroom," I thought. I didn't want Pidgie to get into trouble again, but I didn't want to get into trouble either. Besides, Mom would never kill Pidgie. She might hit her, but she wouldn't kill her. If she got mad enough at me, I was sure she would kill me.

Mom walked into the den carrying the laundry through to the garage. I looked at her pleadingly.

"Don't tell me *you* have to go to the bathroom now," Mom barked, looking exhausted.

"Okay," I said, squeezing my legs together.

When my brother was bad, he got hit too. But he got hit because he was bad—because he broke something or said something nasty to my mother. We all got hit for talking back to our parents, but Frankie never got hit because he had to go to the bathroom.

Although Mr. Jacob, my teacher, was still coming from one to two every day, the school added a new device into my education. It was an intercom directly linked with one of the classrooms. At 9 A.M., I had to report in, like all the other kids. But the school intercom would often be turned off and no one would respond to me. My mother would have to call the principal's office to tell them to turn it on so I could listen. I had to listen to the class until one o'clock, and try to follow along, even though I couldn't see the blackboard and sometimes had no idea what they were talking about. Sometimes, if they were reading out loud, or the teacher was sharing a story, I found it interesting. Mostly, I was bored and would find myself rocking and rubbing my thighs together.

Once in a while the teacher called on me to answer really dumb questions. I didn't realize she was trying to test me. Because Mom was so busy in the morning with my brother and sister, I would often sit in my nightgown while I listened and she would dress me later. I was glad they couldn't see me. Two or three times during the year I was allowed to go into the class for a class party, so I could get to know the children I listened to every day. I longed for contact with them.

A few of the kids who seemed to like me a lot visited me at home or asked me to their houses for parties. One of the boys was named Louis Popp. I liked him a lot too. I thought that if I married him it would be great because my initials would still be C. P.

One Friday night, Dad drove me to Louis' house. He tipped my chair up on the two back wheels and took me down Louis' basement steps. I tried to squeeze my knees together so the kids below me in the basement couldn't look up my flowered party dress, and held tight onto Louis' birthday present sitting on my lap.

"Hi, Connie," chirped Linda. Her hair was teased up around a little blue ribbon.

"Hey, Connie, Lou's mom made great spaghetti," Tom shouted up at me.

I felt myself picking up the rhythm of the rock-and-roll record that was playing. When we reached the playroom floor, Dad said goodbye and patted me on the head. "Have a good time, honey."

I shot him a dirty look. Mom spent a long time fixing my hair just right, and here he was messing it all up. I smiled as Louis walked over to me. "Happy birthday, Louis." The present was too heavy to lift and hand to him, so I glanced down at it and then smiled up at him.

"Thanks," he said, taking the present. "We're playing spin the bottle. Want to play?" He squeezed my hand and whispered, "Sit next to me over in the corner near the cabinet, okay?"

I nodded and he pushed me over to his favorite spot.

"Spin the bottle, Jim," said Donna, a girl with long red braids tied up on top of her head.

Jim, a skinny kid with glasses and his shirt hanging out, gave the soda bottle a good hard spin. When it stopped it was pointing at me. Jim gave me a quick kiss on the cheek. "Do you want me to spin it for you, Connie?" he asked.

"Yeah Jim, go ahead."

Jim spun the bottle and it pointed at me again, which meant that the next boy to my left was "it". Louis smiled and kissed me gently. We both blushed. Louis spun. The bottle pointed at Linda. He kissed her quickly on the cheek.

"Your spin, Linda," offered Louis, handing her the bottle and taking his seat next to me.

Cute Linda with the blue bow in her hair spun hard. The bottle pointed at me when it stopped. I smiled at her and was startled when Louis kissed her on the cheek and took over the bottle. Her cheek looked so soft and warm. I wanted to kiss her cheek too. I didn't know why the rules said that only boys and girls could kiss, but I knew I shouldn't say anything about it.

As the game went on, the bottle pointed to either Louis or me most of the time. I think the floor tilted down towards that side of the basement, which was probably why it was Louis' favorite corner.

According to the rules of the game, you were supposed to switch places with whomever you kissed, but since I was in the wheelchair, that was too much trouble. Louis didn't have any excuse for not moving, except that it was his birthday and his house. He stayed next to me the whole night and we kissed a lot.

The parties were fun, but few and far between. Mom and Dad both tried to fill my life with other activities so I wouldn't be lonely and bored. My parents decided to give me piano lessons. It was very physical for me, kind of like aerobics or mountain climbing. I had to compensate for my muscles being weak and learned ways to make the music sound wonderful by using creative fingering. I dropped off notes I couldn't reach and filled in with other ones that sounded equally good. I could make music!

Besides the piano lessons, Mom taught me to sew and do embroidery. When the Girl Scouts rejected me because I was disabled, Mom started a club with a few neighborhood girls and me. We got together one night a week and learned crafts. Grandma taught me to knit, and she and Mom taught me to cook. Even though I couldn't do much of the physical part, I could follow the steps and learn the recipes.

Dad and I had a lot of fun together. He bought me model kits and helped me make a Morse code set. We went to stockcar races. I used to bet on the cars, and always won. They crashed into each other and everyone clapped when the driver walked away from the car unhurt. They never seemed to get hurt.

"Do you want to go for a ride?" Dad asked one day.
"Okay, where are we going?"

"To the park," Dad responded as Mom came into the room.

"Don't be gone too long, I want to make sure she changes and goes to the bathroom before we eat," Mom explained as she went downstairs to do the laundry.

"Do you want to go flying?" Dad whispered.

"Yeah!" I shouted.

"Shh. Don't tell your mother, or she won't let us go." He swooped me up in his arms and carried me out to the car.

We drove to Zahn's airport and Dad rented a four-seater plane. He strapped me into the seat next to him on a pillow so I'd be high enough to see out the window. He climbed into the pilot's seat and we took off. It was really weird to not be able to walk but to have a father who could fly.

"See, look, there's Jones Beach down there. See the water? See all those cars? That's Sunrise Highway. See? See?" He tilted the plane to the right so I could get a better look. I grinned at him and feasted my eyes on the view. "See, look, there's our house." He circled around with the plane tilted to the right so I could see. "Hi, Mommy," he yelled. Then he chuckled, "She'll never know we're here."

I giggled, "Shh, don't tell her we're here."

When we got home, Mom asked, "Did you have fun at the park?" She took me from my father's arms and we walked towards the house.

"Yeah, it was okay," said Dad, winking at me.

"I had fun," I chirped.

Mom looked at Dad suspiciously. "I heard a plane buzzing around the house an hour ago. That wouldn't have been you two, would it?"

"Oh, Annie, you worry too much!" he chided her.

Mom looked at me. "I don't know," I said. "Ask him."

They bantered back and forth about airplanes and responsibility as I sat patiently on the toilet.

Dad and I also made model airplanes and boats together. Sometimes we went on excursions to the city. He showed me how things were put together, and what various tools were for. I was lucky in that way. Since I had been an only child for a long time, I became his tomboy, even though I was in a wheelchair and couldn't play sports.

Sometimes my dad and Susie's dad took us on adventures like sleighriding. I would invariably fall out of the sleigh, but for the most part, I loved being one of the gang. I couldn't really be sure if I was pleasing myself, pleasing my friends, or pleasing my parents by risking injury trying to do normal things. I went fishing in rowboats, floated in life preservers on lakes, and laid on the grass looking up at the treetops. Once my father propped me up in the crook of a tree limb. It was wonderful. It wasn't the same as trying to ride the rocking horse, because I didn't have to move anything. All I had to do was sit and look around me. It was even better than climbing trees with Susie.

One day, when Pidgie was still an infant, while I was playing the piano, I overheard my mother talking on the phone to the Muscular Dystrophy Association.

"Well, that's very nice of you, but she doesn't have muscular dystrophy."

"Good," I thought to myself since three of my camp friends just died from that. "I wonder what they want?"

"A poster child? I know she's pretty, but isn't she too old?" my mother responded.

I said to myself, "If 'she's' pretty, they must be talking about Pidgie, but what could Pidgie be too old for?"

"Well, thank you very much, I'm sure she'll be very happy." Mom hung up the phone, came in and leaned on the piano smiling at me. "Guess what?"

"What?"

"The Muscular Dystrophy Association has chosen you to be the Long Island poster child. They want you to represent all the children with muscular dystrophy. You get to be in pictures in the newspaper and you may have to go on television. You might even get chosen national poster child for the whole country."

"But I don't have muscular dystrophy, do I?"

"No. The woman from the MDA office said that being a poster child makes many of the kids with muscular dystrophy too tired and sometimes they die sooner because it's too much stress. A lot of the children who are poster children have similar diseases that are not as bad as dystrophy."

I smiled at her while thinking to myself, "I can really walk, but they don't know that. I should do this to help those poor crippled children, because they're really bad off." Out loud I said to her, "I'm glad I don't have muscular dystrophy."

"Me too. Wait until you father hears about all this." She went into the kitchen to make dinner while I finished practicing my piano piece.

While being a poster child, I got to meet many TV and movie stars, judges and other government officials. I learned how to smile and speak clearly. They taught me how to position my body to look appealing, yet evoke compassion. I learned to open my eyes wide for the camera so that I looked more pleading. I learned a great deal about the media and profiteering.

The day before my eleventh birthday, I was on the telethon. I saw a famous entertainer being a tyrant offstage and appearing a martyr on stage. I saw genuine love and giving, and a great deal of hypocrisy. I was appearing as a helpless child who would die if people didn't give enough money, yet I thought I was healthy. I wasn't really a child anymore, yet was supposed to represent all these children. I was expected to be calm and adult in rehearsal, but sweet like a child on stage. It was a long, long day at the studio. I had a big headache driving home in the car. I was very hungry and tired. I was embarrassed because I had forgotten half my lines and had to be prompted. I had to go to the bathroom very badly, but because I had been with my father that day, and he couldn't come with me into the ladies room and I couldn't go into the men's room with him, I had to "hold it" until we got home.

As soon as we got into the house, he lifted me onto the bed so I could use the bedpan. After he lifted me up out of my chair, he acted funny and told me to wait a minute. He went inside to talk to my mother. I heard whispering. Mom came in and told me not to be embarrassed, but that she thought I might have my first period. She put me on the bedpan, and, of course, I was embarrassed. I looked down curiously at myself and saw my pants all full of blood.

I thought of the telethon. Wouldn't the donors be horrified if they knew that I was not a helpless, dying child with muscular dystrophy, but a healthy young woman very much alive? I didn't think that people would want to give money if they knew I had a budding sexuality and could have a long life.

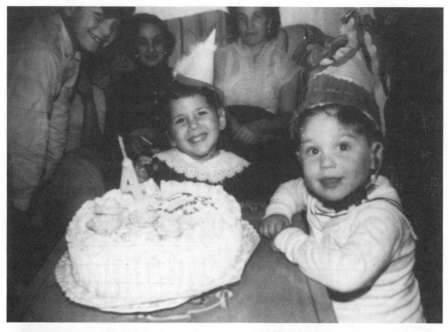

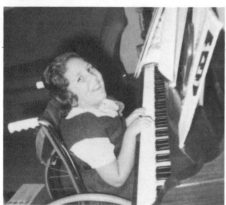

Photos courtesy of Connie Panzarino

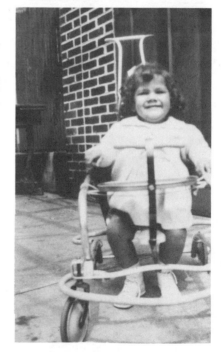

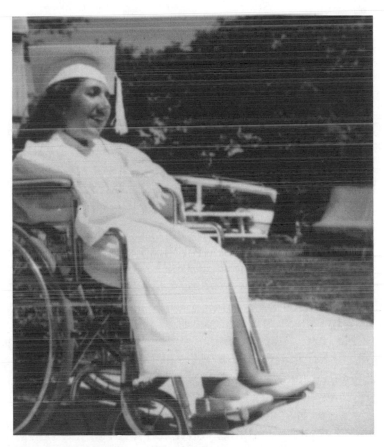

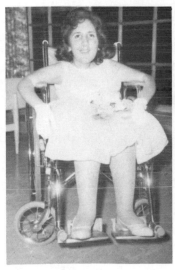

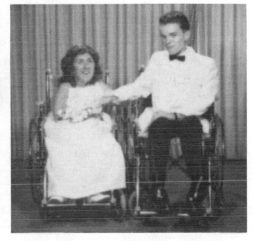

Photos courtesy of Connie Panzarino

6

"JUST HOLD IT"

"Do you think you can *not* go to the bathroom from about seven in the morning until two every day?" Mom asked, standing in the doorway of my bedroom as I sat at my desk reading.

"Why, where are you going?"

"Nowhere. You're going to school, if you can 'hold it' that long. Mrs. Piper is now the head of the nurses' office at Uniondale Junior-Senior High School. Mr. Jacob has been pressuring the school board, Mrs. Piper, and everybody else in town to give you a chance to start seventh grade with all the other kids. He thinks you're too smart to stay home."

My heart began to beat really fast. I could hardly think. "How will I get there?"

"They say they're going to send a special taxi. There's a man named Eddie who owns the company, and he knows how to lift kids like you. You'll only be there half a day, so you can have lunch here when you come home."

"Great! I can hardly wait."

"Well, you don't start for another month or so. I think we'd better go buy you clothes for school."

My parents and my teacher had frequently talked to the school superintendent about my education. I think other parents of disabled children must have discussed the inequity of home education. The school district agreed to try

74

a program at the junior high for me. They said they would allow me to go half days so I wouldn't have to go to the bathroom at school. If it worked with me, they promised they would allow other disabled children to come to school. To me that meant that if I failed, I would fail generations of other disabled young adults.

On my first day of school, Dad brought me into the nurses' office, kissed me goodbye, and left for work.

"Hi, Connie," crooned Mrs. Piper. "This is Mrs. Tomlin, and Miss Rabinowitz, the other nurses here." They said "Hi" and I nodded to each of them. "Your homeroom teacher, Mrs. Murphy, is telling the children all about you, so they'll know what it will be like to have you in class. Every week she will pick one of the other children to be your helper. They will sit next to you, help you with your books and notes and take you to the next class. You will be dismissed five minutes early from each class, so you will have adequate time to get to your next class before the hall gets too crowded. Now, you just wait here until they're ready for you."

"Okay," I said, trying to be patient. I had waited six years to go to school. My stomach was beginning to jump. The nurses' office smelled like a hospital. I wanted to tell her, "No, I want to go to class right now. *I* want to tell the kids about me. What does Mrs. Murphy know about me? She's never even met me." I wondered what it would be like when I got to class.

The phone rang. "All right, Connie, they're ready for you." Mrs. Piper wheeled me down the hall, took me up the elevator, and brought me to my homeroom class. "This is Mrs. Murphy."

I smiled as this young, dark-haired, blue-eyed teacher shook my hand warmly.

"Hello, Connie. Welcome to seventh grade. Class, this is Connie Panzarino. I'd like you all to introduce yourselves to her."

One by one, each child said their name and smiled at me. There were so many of them. I worried that I wouldn't remember everyone's name. Robert, a boy with dark hair and pimples, was chosen to be my first helper.

After English, I went to my history class where I found it difficult to keep my attention on what the teacher was saying. He seemed to say the same thing over and over. Since I had been taught one-to-one at home, I kept responding out loud to him. I didn't know about raising my hand. I couldn't raise my hand very high anyway.

After history, I went to math. My math teacher asked several questions. I knew the answers to all of them. She began to ignore my answers and finally said she didn't want me to answer, she wanted somebody else to answer. I got really mad. If I had the answer, why was she bothering with someone else? I didn't realize that she was trying to make sure other kids understood. I thought the answer was what was important, and if need be we should all figure it out together.

I then went to my science class and loved it. After science, I was taken to the nurses' office. I waited there for my taxi. The nurse put my jacket on because it looked like rain, and then Eddie, the driver, brought me out to the taxi, unstrapped me from my chair, lifted me into the cab, and put my wheelchair in the back seat. There were no safety belts in the cabs in those days. A couple of times on the way home when he stopped short, I slid halfway off the seat.

The teachers had varying reactions to me. Some were a bit condescending. Others were warm and accepting like my homeroom teacher. My English teacher seemed to have a hard time with me. She kept looking at me, but rarely called on me. Halfway through the first quarter, she asked my mother to come in to see her. My mother thought I had done something wrong or that the teacher was going to say that I shouldn't be in school, even though I had received an "A" on my first composition. When my mother went in, the English teacher said that there was nothing wrong, she had no questions, she just wanted to meet my mother and see what she was like. My mother was angry that this woman made her come all the way in to school just out of curiosity.

My science teacher, Mrs. Sullivan, was warm and understanding, and I fell in love with her. When I looked at her, I became all jittery. It reminded me of the way I had reacted to my babysitter, Lois. Mrs. Sullivan was pregnant and had to leave in the middle of the year. I was devastated. I was also jealous of her husband and didn't like the baby that was taking her away from me. To this day I can remember everything she taught me. I still have the notebook.

Everything went well until one day that winter when my friend Janice was pushing me to class. ". . . So then he told me he really liked my hair, but my mother said my hair was too long, so I cut it, but he liked it even though I didn't think he would, so . . ." Janice rambled on as we whizzed down the hall headed toward the elevator.

Just as we were about to pass the door to the teachers' lounge, a big, tall teacher I had never seen before stepped quickly out of the room and turned right into us. He stepped right on my footrest, which acted like a lever and flipped my chair over. He and I both fell to the ground and I landed right on top of his soft round stomach. The chair flipped off to the side and books and papers scattered in all directions. The bell rang and there was a stampede of people in the hall all around us. Janice began shrieking and crying.

"What the . . . are you all right?" The teacher groaned, lifting me off.

I couldn't stop laughing long enough to answer him. I wasn't hurt. Seeing his look of shock and our homework gliding down the hall, I gasped, "I . . . I . . . I'm fine," as he put me into my chair. "Janice, how are you?"

Janice was now laughing and crying. "I'm sorry. I'm okay, I mean, I think I am. Am I going to get thrown out of school? I think we're late for class." She began picking up papers and books.

The second bell rang, and the halls cleared. The teacher wheeled me down to the nurses' office, with Janice trailing behind with her arms full of the debris. I was disheveled, as was the teacher.

Mrs. Piper sent Janice to her class and tried to straighten my clothes and my hair as best she could, then wrote a note home to my parents which said that from now on I had to wear a seat belt on my wheelchair.

The next day, crying, Janice told me that her mother was upset and forbade her to ever help me in school again. Her mother didn't want to take the responsibility. She thought Janice might be sued. I felt like some dangerous thing. I thought this might mean I wasn't allowed to have friends because I was too fragile. But the other kids' moms felt differently about it than Janice's. They still allowed their kids to push me. I felt bad for Janice, because I knew she liked me, and liked helping me.

That first year in school, I fell in love with Glenn. I watched for him every day at ten forty-five from inside my English class as he was on his way to French. If he said "Hi" it made my life feel complete for at least another week. He was a "hood" and liked the "hoody" girls with tight sweaters, short tight skirts, high heels and teased hair. He always wore black pointed boots in true hood fashion, and wore his shirts out, even though wearing untucked shirts was against the school rules. I was a "collegiate." I wore plaid, pleated skirts, loose sweaters, loafers, natural hair and no makeup. Every day I watched him walk by with another girl. Every night I cried and wrote in my diary a description of what Glenn wore, what he said, and my hopes and dreams for our future.

Glenn and I became friends. We did homework together, talked about our Italian families and gossiped about teachers and other kids. He treated me more normally than anyone else did. He taught me how to dance. He would show me the latest dance steps and share the latest popular songs. We both loved the Supremes. He cared about how I looked and advised me how to make my hair look better. He said I was beautiful, but he never asked me out on a date.

Glenn's interest in other girls hurt me, yet he was one of the kindest, most accepting people in my life at that time. We went to nearly all the dances together, but it was never like real dating. I was more of a pal to him. He wouldn't kiss me or let me wear his ring. Every time he said we were just friends, it hurt.

I did fairly well in school that first year, so they allowed another disabled young person to attend. I was proud of myself. I had not failed. I drank as few liquids as possible so that I would not have to use the bathroom. They let me stay another period longer because of my good urinary behavior.

I had no way to hang out with the kids in my classes after school unless my mother or father drove me. It was very hard for them to do that because my mother had my younger brother and sister at home, and my father had his plumbing business. When they did drive me, they had to lift me in and out of the car. By the time I got to a party or other school events, my clothes and hair were disheveled from the lifting and I looked a mess. I was friends with all the girls. We talked about hairstyles and clothes. Instead of saying that I couldn't wear certain clothes because of my physical limitations, I would simply tell them I didn't like those styles. But it wasn't true. I loved straight skirts, and I loved striped sweaters, but they made me look like a big boat. I couldn't hide my big belly that stuck out to the left because of my spinal curve.

Doctors were constantly encouraging my mother to put me on a diet. I couldn't figure out whether I was fat due to my disability, or if I was fat because all the women in my family were fat. I also couldn't figure out whether being overweight impeded my movement or made my disability worse. I thought if I became thinner, the boys might over-look my disability. I even wore a panty girdle for a while even though it sliced into a sore on my side that had developed from my curvature. I had the sore for about five years from wearing tight-waisted clothes. Besides being fat, I was very short, and looked like a child in my chair. I tried desperately to find ways to look more grown-up.

"Linda, how about coming over and listening to records Saturday afternoon?" I asked.

"Sure, that'd be great. Maybe I'll wear my new sweatshirt to show you. It's great. It's tie-dyed."

"Cool. My mom's supposed to take my little brother out, so it should be peaceful."

"Can I come too?" asked Carol, overhearing our conversation.

"Sure."

When Saturday came, we hung out in my room, drinking Coke and playing records. Carol bragged, "I went out last night on a pizza date with Joey, and he kissed me on the cheek!"

"Wow!" I exclaimed. "He's pretty cute. Did he ask you to go steady?"

"No, but I hear Glenn asked you to go steady, didn't he, Linda?" Carol teased.

Linda pulled a ring out of her pocket and opened her hand to show us. "I told him I'd keep it, but I wouldn't wear it yet. We've only been out twice. We're supposed to go to the beach tomorrow with his brother. If things go well, I'll wear it after tomorrow."

My eyes filled up with tears, but I tried to hold them back. "You didn't tell me you went out with Glenn. I like Glenn."

"Let's put on another record." Linda jumped up, ignoring my question.

"Yeah," said Carol. "We shouldn't be talking about this stuff here." She nodded at Linda.

"You wouldn't go out with Joey, would you, Linda? You know that Carol likes Joey, so you wouldn't go out with him if he asked you, would you?"

"That's different, Connie," responded Carol, and Linda nodded agreement. They changed the record, then changed the subject completely.

I realized they thought that since I was physically different, I shouldn't have a boyfriend or even be interested in boys. They never asked me if I wanted to get married or have babies, although they asked each other questions like that all the time. That night I lay in my bed and wept. I played my little transistor radio loudly so my parents wouldn't hear me cry. I couldn't tell them that I wanted to be married some day, because I knew they didn't think anyone would want to marry me. I knew they would say it didn't matter. I fell asleep and dreamed of being married.

I worried about my choice of career. For a while, I wanted to be a piano teacher, but then realized that I wouldn't be able to play complicated pieces or show a person how to play correctly. I decided to be a horse trainer and read all the books in the library about training horses. I gradually began to realize that I was not physically able to be a horse trainer either. I thought about being a famous writer and making lots of money, but I knew writers travelled a lot and

I didn't know if I could do that.

I kept wondering about walking. I started to think that maybe this "not walking" thing had gone on long enough. It was really beginning to interfere with my life. Perhaps I should just make up my mind and decide to walk. I fantasized about it a lot. I knew that everyone would be angry and freaked out if I walked, but I figured that once they got past their initial anger over having catered to me all my life, they would be so relieved that they would forgive me and be happy.

One night when I was twelve my parents decided that they had been neglecting my treatment because they had not been putting me in my braces for about six months.

"I don't want to stand on the braces now. I have to study for a test tomorrow. They probably won't even fit me anymore."

"Don't give your mother a hard time. She's doing what's best for you. You think she likes to put you in those things? It's a lot of trouble, you know," Dad admonished, as Mom buckled all the straps. "I have to take you for your checkup next week. What are the doctors going to say if we tell them you haven't been in the braces since the last time you had a checkup?"

"I don't care about the doctors," retorted Mom, "it's just not good for her to sit all the time."

"Why not? A lot of people like to sit all the time," I protested. "I think sitting is good for me."

"Shut up. Frank, help me get her up."

My father helped swing me up onto my feet. I winced in pain and waited while my legs went numb, as they always did from the tight straps. Mom stood behind me and held me by the waist to keep me balanced. Just then, my three-year-old brother, Frankie, came into the room.

"Connie!" he exclaimed, with delight in his eyes, as he ran

up to me, threw his arms about my waist and hugged me. I put my hands gently on his shoulders and looked down into his eyes. I wanted so much to be a big sister to my brother, like Susie was to her little brother. I had wanted to help *him* learn to walk, yet here he was overjoyed because *I* was standing up. He must have thought I was finally "normal," but I wasn't. Even though I was standing, I couldn't move. When I got back into my wheelchair an hour later, it hurt me to see the disappointed look in his eyes. I wanted to walk for him. I cried that night because I knew I couldn't walk.

I prayed to God that if he wanted me to walk, he should let me walk by the time I was fifteen. I thought that way I could know how to deal with the rest of my life.

The next three years I lived as if when I turned fifteen it would all change. They would discover a cure and I would be well. I figured out the number of hours that I would have to stand to make up for all the sitting I had done. And so, since I would be able to walk at that point, I decided to become a doctor.

Doctors were such a dominant part of my life. Although they did terrible things to me, some of them were kind and sincere. I wanted to be a helpful doctor and not hurt kids. Maybe I could find the cure for my disease and for others too. I didn't think it could be too hard. If I understood at four years old that I couldn't lift my arms, and the doctors all seemed to think I could, then I must be smarter than the doctors. In science class I was learning how bodies work: about bones, muscles and nerves. My disability, I learned, involved problems with nerves. The nerves weren't telling the muscles what to do, so the muscles got weak. It was fascinating to discover the layout of the different systems in the body and how they worked together. My father was a plumber, and he'd lay out plumbing and heating systems and then fix them if there was a blockage somewhere or something didn't flow right. I was sure that's all I needed to have done to me.

I studied long, hard hours. I became close friends with another studious girl named Janet who wanted to be a nurse. We studied a lot together after school. That summer when I was twelve and she thirteen, Janet's family and mine went on vacation together.

"Connie, did you remember to bring your biology kit?" Janet asked as Dad got me out of the car at the summer resort in Connecticut.

"I sure did. I got my microscope, scalpel and a preserved frog. Did you see any moss or algae down by the water that we can check out?"

"Yeah. Let me push you down there and show you the lake." Janet wheeled me around in my chair as my parents unpacked the car. "Let's get my sister, Alice, and see if she wants to come with us."

We spent several days studying the plants and bugs that we found while our parents enjoyed swimming, fishing, and dancing in the dining hall. One afternoon as Janet and I were sitting in the snack bar sipping our Cokes, I suggested, "Janet, don't you think this would be a great place to dissect that frog? There's running water in the bathroom right behind us, a great table, great light and loads of napkins."

"Yeah. What a great idea. I'll go get him. Alice, you stay here with Connie while I get her biology kit, okay?"

"Sure," Alice mused. Alice was ten and very smart, but very dreamy and quiet.

In a few minutes, Janet returned with the kit and we set up our dissection. "You hold it here, Connie, and I'll make the first cut." Janet sliced into the frog and a bunch of formaldehyde ran out. "Quick, Alice, get more napkins."

Alice went to get more napkins from the counter and

came back as we were pinning open the skin of the frog to reveal heart, lungs and various innards we had not identified yet. "People are staring at us," whispered Alice.

"They always stare at me anyway," I retorted.

Janet replied, "Give them something to look at this time, right Conn?"

A man came over and peered at the open body on the table, put his handkerchief over his mouth, doubled over, and went into the men's room. A couple came in, took one look at our project on the table and left.

Janet and I carefully removed the vital organs and put them in little jars. I took notes while Alice kept trying to clean up under Janet's direction.

"What are you kids doing? That's disgusting," snapped a man who had come out from behind the counter. "You can't stay here, you have to leave. Now! I'm going to tell your parents."

"We're going to be doctors," I protested.

"Yes, we're studying," explained Janet.

He threw up his hands and shook his head. "I'm going to tell the director of the resort." He stomped out of the snack bar, leaving customers at the counter. We hurriedly finished the frog and got out of there as fast as we could.

Although I had many friends at school, by the beginning of my freshman year they were beginning to enjoy more and more activities that I could not participate in. Transportation was still a problem, and I found myself dreading the isolation of being homebound on evenings and weekends. My parents planned more and more family outings for us. That helped relieve my boredom, but it increased my feeling of being different from my friends, who went out with their peers.

The next summer, when I was thirteen, I was able to go

back to camp. It meant that for five days a week I could be free from my parents and able to have fun with my disabled peers.

Jack was a fourteen-year-old camper. He had jet black hair and startling blue eyes. One day after lunch, Jack said, "Would you like to go for a walk to look at wildflowers?"

"Okay," I agreed. My skin tingled and my muscles felt jumpy.

Jack wheeled me with his one good hand and pushed me with a swaying gait along the blacktopped wheelchair paths through the camp woods. He struggled to keep my chair straight on the path, since he only had full use of one side of his body. We stopped to look at some flowers and Jack sat beside me on a log.

"You know, Connie, I know that you're Catholic and I'm Jewish, and I don't know if that makes a difference to you, but I really like you. And, I would like very much if maybe I could take you out to dinner for a hamburger or pizza sometime." He was looking down at his feet shyly.

As he turned to look at me, I looked down at his feet too. I swallowed a lump in my throat and whispered, "Yes, I would like that."

We smiled at each other and he walked me back to my afternoon art group. That evening Jack called and explained, haltingly, "My parents said we are too young to go out to dinner. I'm sorry."

The next year Jack died. He had had a brain tumor. That was his disability, and the reason he limped. The kids in camp never knew. He was the first boy to ask me out. I never forgave his parents for depriving us of sharing time together when his life was so short. If Jack had been an able-bodied fourteen-year-old boy in my school we would have been allowed to go out for pizza or hamburgers, but somehow, because we were disabled, there were different rules.

7

HAT IN HAND

When I was about fourteen, I got a phone call from a girl named Maureen inviting me to a meeting with other disabled young adults.

About eight of us, all in wheelchairs and all having some kind of muscle disease, crammed into Maureen's parents' living room. Maureen asked us to introduce ourselves. To my surprise, one of the other kids there was her younger brother. I had thought my family was the only family that had more than one child with a disability.

"I have invited all of you here because you are all disabled like me and we are all teenagers," began Maureen. "Some of us go to special schools, some of us learn at home, and some of us go to regular schools. We all have friends and like to do things that other kids our age do, but it's harder for us to go out without our parents. It's hard to find places to go that are accessible for wheelchairs. Even though I have friends, I sometimes feel very alone because it's hard to go some of the places they want to go.

"Sometimes people have bad attitudes about people with disabilities. People like us make others uncomfortable because they don't understand that this is just the way we are. We don't have to feel bad about it.

"I think we can form a club to go out and do things, and learn about what our rights are, and how we can get what we need. I think we could have a lot of fun together and share a lot of our feelings with each other."

I could feel myself falling in love again. No one had ever talked about these things so clearly before.

"I think it would be a great idea," said Robert, a guy with dark hair and glasses. "Can we go to baseball and basketball games?"

"Yeah," gurgled a voice from a very twisted-up body. "How about a bar, too?"

"Tom, I think we're all a little too young for that, but maybe we could have a party," suggested Chip, Maureen's brother.

Jimmy, a handsome, Irish, sixties radical, asked, "Can we visit some colleges or places where we might be able to work? I'm really concerned with how, and if, I can support myself."

"I'm with you," responded Maureen. "I'm in my last year of high school, and I don't know what I'm going to do yet. Maybe we can form committees on different topics like education or employment and have speakers at some of our meetings."

"I think our biggest problem is going to be transportation," I commented. "Is there anything we can do about that? I mean, my dad drove me tonight, but the whole point is I want to be able to go out even when he can't take me."

"Yeah," said a blond-haired boy from camp named Michael. "We need money to pay bus drivers. Do you think the Muscular Dystrophy Association would give us some money to do that?"

"Well, Chip and I thought about that," replied Maureen, "and we decided that if this is going to be our group, we want to raise our own money because, otherwise, the Association will be telling us where we should go and where we shouldn't go, and what we should and shouldn't do."

"I agree." Tom sipped the soda through a straw in the can that was balanced precariously on his knee. "I think we

should have a rock-and-roll band contest. We could charge
the bands an entry fee and have the playoffs in the audito-
rium of a local high school and charge people to come
watch. Maybe WBAI would play the winning band as a
prize."

"I like that idea, but maybe we need something simple
first, just for some money to set us up to do that," I added.

"Yeah, like a raffle," agreed Michael.

The group got off to a good start. Between the raffle and
the contest we made two thousand dollars. We met once a
month and also planned a monthly outing. We had one or
two able-bodied volunteers helping us with physical tasks.
We went to movies, sports events, dances and even the
World's Fair in New York City.

Through the committees and speakers I learned about Social Security benefits, welfare rights, health insurance, college and job application processes, and government responsibility towards people with disabilities. I was devastated
when I learned that individuals with disabilities were not
covered under the Constitution of the United States or the
New York Bill of Rights. It was legal then for people to ex-
clude other people simply because of disability.

We got letters from people who had been asked to leave
restaurants or hotels because their wheelchairs or bodies
made people uncomfortable. I began to make connections
between the stories I was hearing and what was happening
to me. I started writing letters about it and sending them to
newspapers, friends, relatives, legislators and anyone else
who might read them.

People in stores often stared at or ignored me when I
spoke to them. I remembered when I was eight and my dad
had taken me to St. Patrick's Cathedral. He had parked me
in my wheelchair on the sidewalk near the steps for a few
moments while he went to help a woman carry a baby carriage down the stairs. Since it was windy, he had handed me
his hat and asked me to hold it for him until he came back.

A passerby smiled at me and dropped a quarter in the hat. I was embarrassed and afraid that Dad would be angry at me. By the time he came back, tears of humiliation streaked down my face. Dad picked up his hat and asked me what was the matter. Then he noticed the quarter in the hat. He stared at it for a moment or two, then picked it up and put it in his pocket, smiling at me. "Don't let it bother you. If we stay around here a little while longer, we'll have enough money to go out to dinner." He put his hat on his head and wiped my face lovingly with his handkerchief.

He pulled me up the stairs of St. Patrick's and we went in to tour the church. We put the quarter in the donation box before we left.

Incidents like that or being stared at made me feel awful. Through the young adult group, I did not have to be alone with those feelings. I spent many hours on the phone each day talking to other members. The constant telephone contact made up for the fact that we could only see each other once or twice a month.

In addition to the young adult group, I sometimes attended the Saturday afternoon recreation program at the Cerebral Palsy Association Center. Many of the volunteers from summer camp worked there, and since we, the disabled participants in the program, were in the same age group as the volunteers, many friendships arose between the volunteers and those of us in the program. When volunteers or participants had parties, everyone was invited. For a short time it appeared that my two worlds of friends, able-bodied and disabled, were finally beginning to be integrated.

Then Gary, one of my friends from the young adult group, asked one of the volunteers out on a date. They felt an attraction to each other. The following week, when the Center staff found out about it, the volunteer was told to end the relationship or else she would not be allowed back as a volunteer and would not be given a reference. I think the Center became more and more restrictive about all the volunteers because there began to be more division between volunteers and participants. Although we still had parties together, the teenagers with disabilities would congregate on one side of the room and the able-bodied volunteers on the other. It reminded me of stories of leper colonies and helped me understand what Martin Luther King was talking about.

Because of the separation and because my school friends wouldn't talk to me about boys and sex, I became angry and confused about it all. I didn't know who I was allowed to be attracted to, or if I should be attracted to anybody, but I certainly was turned on by boys. I didn't know what to make of my feelings for Mrs. Sullivan, my science teacher, or Lois, and I wanted to have babies.

One day, Tom, a six-foot-four, gorgeous, blond volunteer at camp, took me in to the pool. He held me with my legs around his waist. I put my arms around his neck to hold on. I liked him. I was fourteen and he was sixteen. I began to feel a bulge between my legs and got very excited but very scared. I had heard of sperm swimming across bathtubs and impregnating women. I liked his bulge with the protection of my bathing suit, but I was afraid being in the water with him might allow the sperm to swim. Just before I got into the pool, I had begun to menstruate. I didn't realize that the cold water from the pool would stop my flow. Since it didn't start again for several days, I was sure Tom had made me pregnant. I was afraid to tell my mother.

I wasn't supposed to get involved with able-bodied volunteers, but if I let myself like a boy with a disability, his parents might prevent us from seeing each other, the way Jack's did. It was also physically more difficult. I could barely lift a fork to my mouth or write with a pen, and the guys with muscle diseases were similar. We couldn't even hug each other.

· · ·

Crash! I looked toward the bushes at the edge of the yard where we were having a Saturday night rock-and-roll party.

"What was that?" I asked Billy. I heard a second crash, followed by a clatter.

"I think that's Jeannie and Doug 'making it' in the bushes," replied Billy, giggling.

"How do they do it?"

"Well, Doug says they both kind of slide out of their chairs onto the ground where they can wiggle over to each other. At the end of the night they'll call out to the volunteers to get them back in their chairs."

I began to wish I had cerebral palsy like they did. "Where's Robert tonight? I haven't seen him for a while."

"Didn't your mother tell you?"

I shook my head.

"You'd better ask your mother." Billy called to ask someone to push him over to get something to drink.

Later that night when I got home, I asked my mother about Robert. She said he had died a month earlier, but she had been told by the Muscular Dystrophy Association that it was better for us kids not to know.

Later that year, Michael died too. I felt the need to go to church, but there were stairs in the church. Uncle Gus, my father's first employer, began sending me Bible study books and pamphlets. They were a great comfort to me.

As young friends died, I began to wonder whether I really did need to worry about a career and a future. At Uniondale High School, we were being encouraged to take aptitude tests and think about what we wanted to be. I just wanted to be. I had had many life-threatening illnesses as a child, and I choked often. I didn't realize until I was in seventh grade that I could die from choking. I went through a ritualized eating procedure for a long time to prevent death. I made a deal with God that if I only ate half of what I was given for a meal, then I wouldn't choke to death. This way, I figured, I reduced my chances of choking by fifty percent. Because I was eating half of everything and was throwing away half of my meal, my mother kept giving me less. The less she gave me, the less I ate, and the less I ate, the less she gave me. I lost weight and my mother told me I was not eating enough. I didn't dare tell anybody what was happening. I kept this up for close to a year, but I liked food. I just decided one day that if I was going to die, I was going to die, so I stopped eating things that I knew I could choke on, like salad or steak. If my mother made salad and potatoes and steak for dinner, all I would eat were the potatoes. Then I started gaining weight because I was eating mostly starches. As friends died and I continued to live, I began to develop a fantasy that I was going to live forever. I just wasn't going to die; I would refuse to die.

That next summer, my parents rented a summer house on the south shore of Long Island. We went swimming, fishing and boating, which any of my high school friends would have envied, but there were no other kids my age there. I had to give up camp, hanging out with Glenn, and talking on the phone with my friends from the young adult group. It was like being in jail on some deserted island. My parents got angry at me for pouting, and said I was unappreciative. But eventually they took pity on me and invited Janet and Alice up for a week.

"Put on *Cruel War*, Janet," I told her, sipping my Coke.

"Okay, Conn." Janet put the record on and leaned back against the cushion to listen. The song played through. Janet asked, "What next?"

"Oh, I don't know. I'm sure glad boys don't get drafted anymore."

"Of course they do, Conn. What are you talking about?" retorted Janet. "Alice, can you get me some ice? Thanks." She handed her glass to Alice, who left.

"No, they don't. They can't. It's not allowed."

"Yes, they do. When boys are eighteen they have to sign up for a draft card. Then if the government needs them to defend the country, they have to go."

I began to cry. "I don't want Glenn to ever be drafted."

"Face it, Conn. It's going to happen."

"No!" I shouted. How could you grow up if grown-ups still fought wars? It was stupid. Glenn was too cute to go to war. "Put on *See You in September*," I told Janet. I lay back in my chair and dreamed about seeing Glenn in September and tried to forget about war.

My fifteenth birthday came and went and I didn't walk. It was then that I fully understood that I couldn't walk. All this time I had been kidding myself. I rejected God for his decision and wouldn't talk to him. I only prayed to the Virgin Mary. I was glad I had chosen the name Bernadette for a confirmation name several years before. Bernadette was a disabled girl who had had visions of the Virgin Mary. Bernadette had dug a stream based on the Virgin's command. The stream had healing waters which healed many people, but it didn't heal Bernadette. The Virgin Mary told Bernadette that she would always be disabled, though she would help heal many others.

I wanted to save others by being a doctor. In my advanced biology class I soon realized that I could not reach the lab counters. No one told me that labs could be adapted for wheelchairs, so I gave up being a doctor. I dropped out of the course, and I decided to be a writer.

My dad's plumbing business was doing better and the two-bedroom house we lived in in Hempstead was just too small for my parents and three kids. My parents bought a house in a wealthier neighborhood in Massapequa. I didn't want to leave Glenn and my other friends. It was terrible. I would never walk, I would never see some of my able-bodied friends again, and one by one my disabled friends were dying. I might as well die too, I thought, as I packed some of my things with my grandmother. Mom and Dad were cleaning and packing in other parts of the house.

My father clanged the radiator cover from the bathroom radiator down on the tile floor. "Ann! What the hell are these things?"

"What?" snapped my mother, walking into the bathroom, "That's funny. They look like little round colored dust balls. I don't know what they are. Just vacuum them up and let's get going."

I could barely breathe. They had finally discovered the thousands of pills I had thrown into the radiator when I was little. I exhaled in relief as I heard the tick-tick-tick of the pills being sucked up into the vacuum cleaner.

8

THE YOUNG ADULTS

My family moved to a big five-bedroom ranch house in Massapequa, on the water, with specially built ramps for Pidgie and me. The church was accessible, the school was accessible, and everyone owned boats. Glenn was jealous. It was hard to leave him. I had kept hoping that he would grow up and marry me in spite of my disability.

I was allowed to stay all day at Massapequa High, except when I had to go to the bathroom. Then they would dismiss me early. But I didn't like the school. All the students were white, and most were Jewish, Irish or Italian. There were two types of students: the "surfer" type and the "collegiate" type. Since I was smart, and in honors classes, I was automatically labelled a "collegiate." Most of the families had a lot of money, and everyone wore a lot of jewelry. I felt out of place, even with three other disabled students in the school. They were much more physically independent than I. They could push their own chairs and looked "normal"— they could pass.

One of them, Wendy, was a beautiful girl. I was envious of her. Her mother got up at five every morning so that Wendy would have at least an hour to put makeup on after spending a half an hour washing her hair. Wendy didn't have a disabled sister. I did. It was difficult for my mother to put me on the toilet several times a day and wash and dress me every day, let alone to wash my hair more than once a week. It was odd to not be the only "special" one in school. Besides Wendy, there was also a girl in a wheelchair named Darlene. She could not only stay the whole day without going to the bathroom, she often stayed after school, too. She barely ate so she would look thin and attractive to the boys. Wendy and Darlene were unresponsive when I said there should be a way for me to go to the bathroom at school. They were too concerned with seeming "normal" to acknowledge bodily needs. The other disabled student in the school, John, was a freshman who had had polio as a little kid. Bathrooms weren't a problem for him because he could just pull his thing out, aim and shoot. I wished I could.

I tried to make friends with some of my able-bodied peers. I made sure to be open and friendly. I finally made a friend named Barbara, a tall, quiet young woman a year younger than me who lived down the block. We went to football and basketball games together. I tried to make friends with other kids when we were at the games, but it was hard. Barbara was shy, and I had no independent mobility.

There was a good-looking boy with brown hair and hazel eyes who I ran into a lot in the hall while I waited for my special mini-bus. He usually wore wrestling team shirts. When I said "Hi" to him, he would say "Hi" back, although he never looked me in the eye. He wasn't aloof towards me like I felt the other kids were, just shy. I went to some wrestling matches and found out he was one of the star wrestlers on the team and that his name was Ron Kovic. The next time I saw him in the hall, I called out, "Hi, Ron!" His response was an embarrassed smile and then a nod.

I was angry at my parents for moving me so far away from my friends. I figured they had moved because they had made money and wanted to live in a higher class neighborhood. But we could have bought a larger house in Hempstead that would have met the family's needs. Living on the water and having a boat didn't make up for losing my friends.

I hated the new house, my family, and my new life. I couldn't separate out any of it. My parents grew angry at me for being ungrateful. I didn't care. I wanted to die. My only link with my past life and friends in Hempstead was the telephone, and it was too expensive to use. Glenn came to visit once in a while. I never saw Susie anymore. She had developed epilepsy around the same time that our parents had had a big fight. We hadn't been seeing each other too often in Hempstead anymore, and now the distance made it impossible.

The disabled young adult group became my lifeline. There were a few people nearby I could talk to on the phone for free. I lived for the monthly meetings. I held the offices of treasurer, vice-president, then president.

My friend Barbara became a babysitter for my sister and brother. It was my job to supervise her while she was babysitting, since I was a year older than she was. We had fun doing it together. A friend of hers raised poodles. I wanted one but knew that my mother would never agree, so I didn't even ask them. I visited each litter of puppies. There was one fluffy little beige one that I mooned over.

One night when Barbara was babysitting my brother and sister, I decided to try doing a painting of the puppy from memory. Long after Frankie and Pidgie were asleep, I finally asked Barbara to help me clean up.

"Barbara, I think I'm done for the night. Can you clean up these brushes and put my painting away?"

"Sure, Conn. Wow, that looks great. It looks just like that puppy you like." Barbara picked up the palette, which was full of excess paint. "What should I do with this?"

I looked at her and at the paint, then stuck my index finger in the yellow. I began smearing it on the tray-table that I was working at. Barbara giggled, took some red paint on her finger and joined me.

"Have some paint, Barb," I said, smearing some on her arm.

"Thanks, Conn, here's some for you." Barbara put two red dots on my cheeks. Then she put some on her own nose.

"This is crazy!" I exclaimed.

We began laughing hysterically and smeared paint on each other and ourselves. It took an hour of hard rubbing and a lot of turpentine to clean us both up, but we had a good time. When we were done, I signed my painting "Chettie," short for Concetta.

Two months later, at Christmas, I began taking little gifts out of my stocking. I pulled out a dog bone, a leash and a blue rhinestone collar. "What is this?" I thought to myself. "Is Dad playing a joke on me, like the year he put coal in the bottom of our stockings?" I looked up to see a ball of white fluff tumbling into the den.

"It's for you, Connie. Isn't he cute?" My mother picked up the little poodle and put him on my lap.

I sobbed into the puppy's fur, and he began licking my face. I had thought my parents hated me for my ungratefulness, and yet they gave me this wonderful gift. I felt I didn't deserve it. I loved the puppy. I named him Bobo. He grew into a soft, white, fluffy poodle. He helped fill my loneliness, and he helped me forgive my parents.

One of the places that the kids often went was the library. Since it was way across town, I couldn't meet them there unless my parents drove me. When I got word that the town was building a new library just a few blocks from my home, I was ecstatic. I loved to read. If there was a library so close, I could be wheeled there by a friend.

Towards the end of my first year at Massapequa High, the new library was completed. To my dismay, there were over a dozen steps at the entrance, making it totally inaccessible to me. My disappointment quickly turned to rage, and I called the library.

"Hello. My name is Connie Panzarino. I would like to know when your next board meeting is?"

"Let's see, oh yes, it's on Wednesday, June eighteenth at 8 P.M. in the board room in the basement of the library," replied the woman who answered the phone.

"Thank you. I would like to discuss the inaccessibility of the library at that meeting. Is there anyone I can talk with to get that arranged?"

"Yes, I will talk to the chairman and see if he can put that on the meeting agenda."

"Also, I'd like to mention that I'm in a wheelchair, and I would like to come to the meeting with several other friends who may be in chairs too. Is there anyone who can help get us in since there isn't a ramp?"

There was a pause. "I will have to check with the chairman on that. May I have your number so he can call you back?"

I gave her the number. Several days later the chairman called and said that he and the other trustees would be happy to assist in carrying us downstairs to the basement.

I immediately got on the phone to people from the young adult group, the Muscular Dystrophy Association, a nearby nursing home, and the Association for Better Conditions for the Disabled (ABCD). I got five adults in wheelchairs to go with me to the board meeting. All of them were big, heavy people, the heaviest I could find. Then I called the local newspaper and asked them to cover the meeting because it was going to deal with a very important issue.

The night of the meeting we all assembled outside the rear library door that went to the basement.

"Dad, could you go down and tell them we're here, please." Dad went down the stairs and came back up, followed by seven or eight middle-aged and older men in business suits. They introduced themselves to each of us.

"How can we help?" offered the chairman.

"Well, sir," replied Roy, a large, middle-aged man from ABCD, "we need you to carry us down the stairs, unless there's another entrance with a ramp."

"No problem," said one of the other trustees. "Just show us how to do it." He looked at my father.

"Don't look at me," Dad replied. "I have a bad back. I can help carry her down, she's my daughter, but I'm afraid these guys are too heavy for me." Dad winked at me and tipped me up on my back wheels and bounced me gently down the steps. The man from the local newspaper began snapping pictures.

Dad and I sat in the conference room and waited to the sound of a great deal of thumping, panting and groaning. One by one the people in wheelchairs rolled into the room. We smiled at each other and remained quiet. Several more of the trustees took off their jackets and ties, hung them on chairs and went out to help carry more people down. Dad leaned over to me and whispered in my ear, "Wait'll they have to carry everybody up again."

After about half an hour, the trustees assembled and ran their usual business meeting. The last item on the agenda was the inaccessibility of the library.

"Is there any need to discuss the fact that we must make this library accessible, gentlemen?" the chairman addressed the other trustees.

"No," chorused the trustees.

One trustee added, "I move that we make this library accessible immediately."

"I second," said another.

"All those in favor?" called out the chairman.

"Aye," they chorused.

"Opposed?"

Silence.

"Abstentions?"

Silence.

"This board has now voted to make this library fully accessible as soon as possible. Meeting adjourned."

Everyone clapped and I shouted "Hurray!" since I couldn't clap very loud. We all shook hands. Dad and I left. We could hear the grunts and groans behind us as we walked home.

"Congratulations, hon," Dad patted me on the shoulder.

Four months later, the woman from the library called. "The chairman of the Board of Trustees of the library would like to invite you to the opening of the new ramped entrance to the library. It will be this Sunday at 2 P.M. He would like to know if you and your friends could come a little earlier so we could take some publicity pictures."

"Yes." I said, triumphantly. "It will be an honor to be there."

That Sunday there were about thirty people at the base of the library ramp. The men from the Board of Directors all shook hands with those of us who were disabled. The mayor gave a ten minute talk, and the local newspaper took pictures of me and the other disabled people going up and down the ramp.

When I got home, I called Jimmy, from the young adult group, to share my victory. He was becoming quite a radical activist himself. He was four years older than I, and he was attending the community college. Jim was excited about the library ramp. He told me he had just joined SDS—Students for a Democratic Society. He wouldn't tell me much more over the phone, just something about how if the millionaires were made to live like the rest of us there would be plenty of money to go around and nobody would be poor.

I was beginning to like Jim the way I liked Glenn. He'd been complimenting me a lot on the way I looked and on things I did. At the end of one young adult meeting, while we were hanging out waiting for the vans, he sang "When

Irish Eyes Are Smiling" to me in his beautiful Irish tenor voice.

At the next young adult group meeting, Jim sent me a note which said, "Meet me at the phone booth during break, okay?"

I looked at him and nodded.

Since I couldn't wheel my own chair, and Jim could barely wheel his, we could never really be alone. I asked one of the volunteers to wheel me to the phone and leave for fifteen or twenty minutes. My heart pounded as I waited for Jim to slowly wheel himself to the phone. I had never been kissed on the mouth by a boy before. Now might come the big moment. I was anxious, excited and scared.

Jim finally came. We talked. He winked at me, and I blushed. He took my hand. All of a sudden he leaned over and kissed me on my mouth. It was so hard and so fast, he knocked me off balance and my head fell back. I couldn't lift it up again and neither could he, so we had to wait for the volunteer. It was awful! I was so embarrassed I wanted to die. The next time Jim kissed me, and all the times after that, he put his arm around me first, to give support. Practice makes perfect.

My mother hired a housekeeper named Carol. She was a young spunky woman in her twenties from Antigua. I grew to like her a lot, and she became my buddy. She would carry me upstairs to her room and show me pictures and how to curl hair.

She was the first person I remember who encouraged me to have relationships. If she was babysitting my brother and sister, and I wanted to be with Jimmy, she would make sure that we had time alone. She could lift me and drive the family car, and she took me to get ice cream, or to a movie when she had the time. It was a new-found freedom to be able to go out "alone," without my family or a large group like the young adult group. It was great.

A few times I noticed that people on the street were staring at Carol instead of me, and sometimes being downright rude to her. I slowly realized that this was because she was black. I started taking more interest in the Civil Rights movement, and feeling more respect for what Jimmy and his friends in SDS were talking about.

When she had been there about three months, my mother started fighting with her about money and the quality of her work. I think at first my mother had appreciated having help, so when Carol first came everything she did was fine. After my mother had had a break for a while, she began to want to do things her way again. My mother had had two previous live-in housekeepers. One was an older Scottish woman, and the other was a Panamanian woman. Neither of them had lasted more than three months either. The arguments between Carol and my mother felt familiar, except that while I hadn't become particularly attached to either of the first two housekeepers, I was very attached to Carol.

Late one afternoon, their fight ended in tears. Carol ran upstairs and my mother ran into her bedroom. I heard her talking loudly to my father on the phone. I sat in the kitchen feeling helpless and hungry. I hadn't had dinner yet. Frankie and Pidgie were watching television.

Carol came into the kitchen, carrying her suitcase. "This has nothing to do with you, you know. You're a really good kid." She put her house key on the kitchen table, squeezed my shoulder and then left through the back door.

Mom came in a few minutes later. "Well, now that that bitch is gone, maybe we can have a nice dinner together for a change." She hugged me and began setting the table. "She treated me like I worked for her! Don't you think that was terrible?"

"Yes," I said. I was afraid that if I didn't take my mother's side, she might hit me. I wanted to cry, but there was no way for me to go into my bedroom. I thought back to the two months before Carol came, when my mother was screaming and yelling at all of us. I remembered her hitting me repeatedly in the face, saying it was all my fault when she dropped a bottle of milk she'd taken out of the refrigerator. I didn't want that anymore. I didn't know whether to be angry at my mother for firing Carol, or angry at Carol for leaving. My mother really needed her.

"Hey, Conn, how're you doing? Hey, Annie!" Dad burst into the room, his arms full of packages, the newspaper and his jacket. They gave each other a long drawn-out kiss.

"Oh, it's so good to be alone again, isn't it?" Mom sighed, looking into his eyes.

"Sure is, Annie." Dad looked over at me. "That bitch stole one of your mother's checks and tried to cash it at the bank. Can you imagine that, trying to steal from your mother! It's a good thing the bank called." He looked at my mother. "You let her off easy. I would have called the cops."

I didn't know who or what to believe. I felt sorry for my mother, sorry for Carol, and most of all, sorry for myself.

After a few months, Mom hired a young mother's helper. It lightened the strain on her, but it didn't help during the night when she had to get up periodically to turn or toilet my sister and me. Sometimes my father got up to do it, but he couldn't hear us himself. He had tinnitus from flying on bomber runs in World War II. The constant ringing in his ears made him hard of hearing. My mother always had to wake him up when we called, which meant that she would wake up anyway. Seventeen years of constantly broken sleep had to have affected her. She would get so crazy from being woken up so much in the middle of the night that she would scream at me and scratch me or move me roughly. I know she didn't mean to, and she felt terrible afterwards, but I figured the only way out for her was for me to eventually move out. I wondered if I would ever be able to find a job and afford someone to take care of me so I could live on my own.

Life with my family was complicated by the conflicting needs of myself and my sister, both in wheelchairs, and my very active younger brother. Our arguments seemed endless, a way of life.

Early one evening, I was studying for a French test in the den to the sound of Frankie and Pidgie watching Bugs Bunny cartoons on TV. Mom yelled to Frankie, "Bring your sisters in."

Five-year-old Pidgie screamed, "What are we having, Mom? Macaroni?"

"What a dope," snapped seven-year-old Frankie, wrinkling his nose. "That sure doesn't smell like macaroni."

"Food," came the reply.

"What kind of food?" Pidgie crowed.

"Shut up!" Frankie yelled. "I can't hear the TV."

"You're supposed to turn it off and bring us in, Frankie," I said. He pretended not to hear me. "Frankie. Listen to me," I insisted.

"Okay, okay! I know. You don't have to yell," he shouted as he snapped off the TV and slammed the cabinet doors.

As Frankie carefully wheeled Pidgie up the step and into the kitchen, she nagged, "Frankie! Be careful and don't tip me."

"Ugh! Pidgie's getting fat." I could hear him groaning and bumping her chair into the table leg as he tried to position it.

Frankie came into the den to get me.

"Put my feet up first. *Devenir*—to become. *Devenir, devenir.* Frankie! I said put my feet up first. *Je devenis, tu devenis, il*— Ow! Watch it before I clobber you," I yelped, still mumbling my French.

"You wish," he taunted. He backed me away from my study table and started pushing me quickly into the kitchen.

"Slow down!"

He poured on the speed. "Here we come!"

"Frankie! Be careful with her. I told you not to run with the wheelchairs," scolded Mom.

"Where's Daddy?" I asked. "Mom, aren't you eating with us?"

"He's coming home late again," answered Mom as she cut up the steak on my plate into bite-sized pieces. "I'll wait and eat with him." She finished fixing my plate and began to cut up Pidgie's steak and broccoli.

Frankie sat down at his place and began cutting up his own steak. I interrupted him. "Frankie, get the catsup." He got up to get the catsup, brought it back to the table and picked up his knife and fork. "Frankie, hold your knife in your right hand," I ordered. He gave me a dirty look. "Mom, you forgot the milk. Patricia! Stop rocking back and forth. Do you want to have your brakes locked?"

"Connie. I . . . I . . . I can't help it, but . . . ."

"Patricia, do you have to go to the bathroom?" asked Mom sternly.

"Well, will I have to go to bed if I go now?" she asked, blinking her big brown eyes.

"Can you wait until after supper?" asked Mom.

"No," came the reply.

"Come on, Miss," snapped Mom, putting down the milk bottle. She took Pidgie away from the table and wheeled her to the bathroom.

"She does the same thing every night. Why doesn't she go before everyone sits down?" I wondered. "Frankie, sit up straight and pour the milk." He got up again and filled the three glasses, knocking over the salt in the process.

Mom came back in with Pidgie after several minutes and sat her at the table. "Is everything set now? I'm going to go in the den and read the paper while I wait for your father. Now stop arguing." She walked out of the room.

Frankie picked up his fork and was just about to take

a bite when Pidgie and I yelled in unison, "Grace!" He dropped his fork, and steak juice splattered all over his shirt. I shot him a disapproving glance. "Go ahead, Pidgie," I ordered.

"Bless us Lord... Bzz... Bzz... Amen."

Frankie looked down at his plate and said, disgustedly, "Broccoli!"

"Frankie, it won't kill you," chirped Pidgie.

"Pidgie, leave him alone and eat your meat," I said, defending him. "Please push my milk closer, Frankie; I can't reach it."

"Sure," he said. "Having a test tomorrow, Conn?"

"*Oui, oui,*" I replied.

"Connie, you shouldn't say piggish things," scolded Pidgie.

"That's French, stupid," said Frankie.

"Patricia! Shut up, and eat your meat," I barked. "And you," I glared at my brother, "eat your broccoli."

"Aren't they eating?" yelled Mom from the den.

"Frankie finished everything but his broccoli, and Pidgie ate everything but her meat," I reported.

"Pidgie, why are you rocking?" Frankie asked innocently.

She was startled. She looked guiltily at me and said, "Connie, I... I can't help it, but... do you think I have to go to the bathroom again?"

"Well, if you don't know if you have to go, how am I supposed to know?" I demanded.

"Well, I think I do, but... Can I go?"

"No!" shouted Mom from the den. "Stop bothering Connie and eat. Both of you."

"Frankie," I whispered, "eat two bites of broccoli, and Pidgie, you eat three more pieces of meat, and we can throw the rest away and go inside."

"Aye, aye, Captain," Frankie said as he washed the broccoli down with his milk. Pidgie ate three pieces of cold dried-up steak.

Pidgie and I yelled in unison, "Take me to the den!"

"Sure, Conn," he said. "I'll be right back for you, Pidgie."

"Okay," she agreed, not having much choice in the matter. He put me back at my table in the den, brought Pidgie into the room, and turned on the TV. Mom got up and went to the kitchen to clean up.

"Frankie, you can't put the TV too loud, because Connie's studying," said Pidgie sweetly.

"If you'd shut up, she'd be able to study," Frankie barked.

"Both of you! Shut up!" I screamed.

There was a knock at the den door. It was Daddy. Frankie opened the door and everyone yelled, "Hi, Dad."

"Mommy's in the kitchen," Pidgie informed him.

He nodded and went into the kitchen.

"You're late again," Mom snapped at him. They began arguing.

I concentrated harder on my studying and began to say my French words out loud. As the volume of the argument increased, I drifted off into a fantasy about becoming rich and moving out on my own. In my mind, I considered different vocational scenarios. I was a piano teacher who became a horse trainer who went to veterinarian school and became a researcher and wrote a book and married a scientist. The house became quiet and I settled back into my studying. I knew I needed good grades to do any of these things.

One day, early in my senior year, I was called down to the guidance office in school to meet with a man from the Office of Vocational Rehabilitation Commission (OVR). He said that OVR could help pay for my college education. I told him I wanted to be a writer because I felt that was something I could do no matter how disabled I became. He arranged for ten hours of psychological and aptitude testing. When I took the tests, I knew I would score very high in the sciences, since I had once wanted to become a doctor and had had an interest in science. I deliberately answered all the medical and science questions wrong, forgetting that I also studied my math so that I could be a doctor. I therefore scored super high in math, a subject that I had no interest in.

After the testing, he said I should be a mathematician. He told me that I had no aptitude for writing. He also told me that perhaps I had an aptitude for working with people as a social worker, but that according to the psychological testing, I was too emotionally unstable to do that kind of work. I thought to myself, that's no surprise: I was drinking insufficient fluids in order not to have to use the bathroom in school; I was eating mostly starches, because I could not safely swallow meats; and I was needing to fight every day to get my physical needs met. It was no wonder the tests showed some instability.

The OVR counselor asked, "Think you can manage in college?"

"Yes," I replied.

"Well, how will you type your term papers?" he challenged.

"I don't know. Probably slowly."

"How will you go to the bathroom?" he taunted.

"I never went to the bathroom in high school," I retorted. "So why should I have to go to the bathroom in college?"

"How will you get from class to class?"

"I'll ask the other students to push me the way I've been doing in high school."

He never suggested Vocational Rehabilitation providing me with an attendant while I was in school. He was not supportive. Jimmy later told me that OVR often paid for people to read for, write for, or feed disabled students at the community college.

"Well, I think we could help you with tuition if you agree to become a mathematician. Think about it," the counselor said, snapping the lid on his briefcase.

The next day I called the local newspaper. "Hello, my

name is Connie Panzarino. I'm a disabled senior at Massapequa High School. I belong to a young adult group for teenagers with disabilities. I'd like to know if you'd be interested
in a monthly column on the activities of the group. I think it
might help educate a lot of people."

Within a few days, the paper hired me as a volunteer col-
umnist. Three months later, I sent my OVR counselor a
copy of the three monthly columns that had been published, a short story I had published in my high school liter-
ary magazine, and a copy of the last letter I had received
from him. His letter had stated that I did not have the aptitude to be an English major. His letter was quite ungram-
matical, so I had taken the liberty of correcting it with a red
pen. I was determined to show him just how "emotionally
unstable" I could be.

Several weeks later, I received a letter from my OVR
counselor stating that I was approved as an OVR candidate
for college. That meant that they would pay my full tuition
and books, and I could major in English.

Glenn and I remained friends even after I moved. Sometimes when my parents went out, he and I would babysit for
my younger brother and sister. A few times when they
stayed out exceptionally late, we lay in bed together, close
and warm, and went to sleep. I became excited, but we were
never openly sexual. He denied the sexually provocative
things we did and always said we were just friends. My parents denied my sexuality too. Once when my mother
"caught us," she asked Glenn what he was doing.

"Sleeping," he said.

She just said, "Oh well, we're home now so you can sleep
upstairs if you want to." Mom never left the house if Glenn
and a girlfriend of mine were there at the same time because
something might "happen" between them. I was her daughter, but strangely enough she didn't seem at all concerned

that something might happen between Glenn and me.

High school graduation came as a sad and scary event for me. Graduation was supposed to mean adulthood and responsibilities, yet I was still physically helpless. Because I could not wheel myself and because the procession went up and down steps, the school administration directed my father to park me in my chair out on the empty football field to await my classmates. I sat there alone in the hot sun for an hour before the procession was complete. I was eight feet to the side of the first row so I could not whisper comments or share in the jokes the girls were telling. Each graduate walked up and across the stage to receive their diplomas. When my name was called, the principal came down to me and shook my hand. As I was struggling to hold the diploma, I wondered what I would do with it in the future.

9

THE BLACK HOLE

In 1965, I applied to the State University at Stony Brook and was rejected because I was disabled. The rejection letter said, "It is unrealistic for a disabled person to expect to go to college." The campus was architecturally accessible, but they still didn't want me.

I then applied to Hofstra University, which was not wheelchair accessible. I had heard that they were beginning the second program in the nation that openly accepted qualified disabled applicants. I was one of the first five disabled students accepted. Dr. Yuker, a psychologist with cerebral palsy, spoke to my freshman class about attitudes toward the disabled. He spoke with slurred speech, his face contorted with muscle spasms. He talked about civil rights, the right to be autonomous, and about where people's negative attitudes came from and what could be done about changing them. I savoured each word he said and imprinted them in my mind.

The physical reality of attending classes was often difficult. Since I could not wheel my manual chair, I hitched rides back and forth across the campus and up and down stairs with passing students. I would have the previous helper park me in a well-trafficked thoroughfare or at the bottom of the stairwell. Then I would smile and try to catch people's eyes. If someone offered help who did not appear strong enough, I would explain what I needed and ask them to find some people who could help them. It always took two people to get me up and down the stairs.

Usually when I asked someone, they were willing to help. But sometimes students would be in a hurry or be afraid to help. I didn't let them off the hook very easily. If they said "No," I would ask them, "Why not?" If they said they were afraid, I would ask them what they were afraid of. If they were afraid of making a mistake or hurting me, I would explain that I would be able to tell them what I needed and that I wouldn't hold them responsible if something happened. I began to write about their reactions in my writing class. I was educating hundreds of people a month about disability just by asking them for help.

Sometimes I got tired of it. It was a relief when students on campus got to know me and other disabled students and were able to offer a lift or a push with expertise. Soliciting for help took a lot of time and energy. As a result, I was often late for class. It was difficult to have to wait out in the rain or snow for a push. I dreaded the bad weather because people's shoes became slippery, and it became even more dangerous to be taken up and down steep stairs in my wheelchair.

Special wheelchair van transportation cost twenty dollars per hour, which amounted to eighty dollars per day. We couldn't afford it, so when my father couldn't drive me, I took taxis back and forth to campus. Sometimes when the taxi drivers saw me waiting in my wheelchair, they wouldn't stop. Once I sat in the rain for over an hour while three different taxis passed me by. I got soaked. The cab drivers did not know how to lift me or fold my chair and put it in the trunk. I had to explain each time. Since there were no seat belts in the cabs, I prayed all the way home that we wouldn't stop short. At times I slid part way out of the seat, but I never landed on the floor. I could only see the tops of the trees and the telephone poles as I slouched there in the front seat. I had to direct the driver the twenty miles to my house using these as guides.

One time the cab driver lifted me into the cab, turned around to fold my chair, and recoiled oddly from the chair before he continued following my directions to remove the cushion and fold the wheelchair. I felt something ooze between my legs. "Damn it!" I thought. "My period. I bet I bled through onto the cushion again. I am probably drenching the seat of the cab in blood." There was absolutely nothing I could do but pretend everything was just fine.

Once I had diarrhea at school. I had to hold it in for two hours until the cab came, and then during the whole ride home. I was sick for two days after that. There was an infirmary and nurses on campus just as there were at the high school and the grade school. But, just as at my previous schools, the college nurses wouldn't take responsibility for toileting me. Often when I needed to go to the bathroom, I would tell myself I didn't really have to. After all, my mother had said that to me many times. If I needed to go to the bathroom two hours after I had already gone, she would often say, "You just went two hours ago, you can't have to go now." I thought there was something wrong with my mind. After being contradicted so many times, I didn't trust my own sense of reality.

Glenn and I were still friends during college, although he went to a different university. I asked him to take me to a ball at Hofstra. We danced and had fun. Drinks were included in the tickets, so Glenn drank more than usual. I had to help him drive me home. I told him how to steer and when to stop. We drove home about ten miles an hour. It took us an hour and a half. When we got home, he got out of the car and threw up in the canal behind my parents' house, then took me inside. I was afraid that if my parents found out, they wouldn't let me go out with him.

Glenn was jealous of my other relationships. He would encourage me to be friends with people, and go out and do things, but then would get over-protective and say, "I don't think you should go and hang out with so-and-so that much, I don't like them." If he had been my boyfriend and wanted to tell me not to see someone, I might have listened, but he was only my friend. He acted like he owned me, and that reminded me of my mother. But, being owned by him seemed better than being owned by my mother because he never hit me. He protected me. When we were at a party, if I started choking, he was beside me in a second. If somebody was dancing with me, and my head fell back, he was right there to lift it up. It was as if he knew what I was feeling.

One afternoon after lunch, we were talking while Glenn did the dishes.

"You think you'll ever get married, Glenn?"

"Oh, yeah. But first I want to have enough money for a big house and a car."

"I want to get married, too," I said cautiously. I knew I wanted him to marry me. Then he could really own me.

Glenn stopped washing the dishes and turned off the water. He sighed and turned to me, his eyes filled with tears. "If I love you as much as I do, and can't marry you, I don't think anyone will ever be able to marry you." He went back to washing the dishes.

He had just admitted that he loved me, but wouldn't marry me. What if he was right that no one else would want to either? I felt my stomach sinking and fought back bitter tears.

Soon after, I became very ill. I knew I was very ill, and so I kept talking on the phone to my friends so I wouldn't feel alone. Part of me was scared I would die, and part of me didn't care anymore. My mother thought I wasn't that sick because I was talking on the phone.

Uncle Pete, my father's brother who worked in a hematology lab, came to visit because he'd heard I was ill. He saw how pale I was and realized I was pretty sick, but he didn't want to alarm me or my parents.

"Let me do a blood count on you, all right Conn? Just for the hell of it."

"Okay, you bloodsucker."

"Yeah, that's me! I've been doing this to you since you were born. Let me get my bag in the car. I'll be right back."

I lay back and closed my eyes. I felt like I was falling into a long dark hole. I jerked my eyes open. Uncle Pete was back already, quickly taking things out of his bag. He was moving very fast. He took my hand, stuck my finger with the little jabber he used and put some of my blood into a little tube. "See you later," he said as he put everything in his bag, snapped it shut and hurried out of the room.

I heard mumbling in the hallway and then my mind wandered off. About twenty minutes later, Mom came in. "Your Uncle Pete called and said we have to take you to the hospital right away. He's going to meet us there in the emergency room. He said your blood count is very low and you need blood right away. He said we shouldn't even take time to dress you."

Dad lifted me into my wheelchair, pajamas and all, and they wrapped a blanket around me. On our way out the door we passed Ruth Mayorga, a neighbor, in the kitchen. She had come over to take care of my sister and brother.

In the emergency room, I learned that my hemoglobin was 1.8, 5 points below the level where I should have been unconscious. They rushed me into the X-ray room and then back to the emergency room, where two doctors argued at the foot of my stretcher. One said that there was nothing they could do, nothing showed up on the X-ray, and I was evidently hemorrhaging internally from some unknown complication of my disability.

The other doctor insisted that I must have a hidden stomach ulcer, since ulcers were prevalent on my father's side of the family and since I had been vomiting and passing blood at home. The first doctor argued that transfusions and extensive treatment would be a waste of time and money, since I was disabled and going to die anyway. The second doctor argued that a transfusion really wasn't that expensive, and that antacids, jello and milk were not considered extensive treatments, and that he would be more than willing to take responsibility to try that for a week.

Each time I closed my eyes I sank deeper into the black hole. The last time I went into the hole there was a bright light at the other end. I fought hard to open my eyes and was relieved to see Doctor Number Two smiling down at me. He had won the argument and was preparing my transfusion. They put me in a room next to a woman who had slashed her wrists. I thought to myself, "Why would anyone like her want to do that to themselves?" I felt a twinge of nausea and realized that my ulcer was a more passive form of the very same thing, only internal. The next day, the nurse told me that if my uncle hadn't come over when he did and gotten me to the emergency room, I would have been dead by morning.

The doctor said I needed to reduce stress in order to heal my ulcer. My parents stopped yelling for a while. Glenn bought me a gold bracelet to always remember our "special" relationship. I think he felt guilty after I nearly died. OVR agreed to provide special transportation to and from school, which eliminated the stress of taking taxis. I transferred to a smaller division of Hofstra that was physically more manageable for me. It greatly reduced the number of times I needed to be pushed across campus or pulled up and down

steps. All of the classes for New College were in two build-
ings, one of which had a ramp. Following doctor's orders, I
ate baby foods and gave up Coke that year, and my ulcer
healed.

Although the new transportation was physically easier
because I could ride in my wheelchair, I had less control of
the scheduling. I would get dropped off at Hofstra at 6:45 or
7 A.M. even though my classes didn't start until eight-thirty.
The only building open at that time of the morning was the
Student Union, and they didn't start serving breakfast in the
cafeteria until seven. So I'd sit in the hall until seven, catch a
push from one of the cafeteria workers into the cafeteria,
and wait for my friend Tom to get up and have breakfast. I
would get anxious when he was late. If he didn't come down
by seven-fifteen, I would have somebody push me to the
pay phone.

Once morning I called to wake him up. "Are you coming
down for breakfast today?"

"Breakfast? Oh yeah, breakfast. Well yeah, I think maybe
I could consider coming down for breakfast. I'll be right
there." Tom rushed right down and met me by the phone.
"I'm sorry I was asleep." He rubbed his eyes. His hair was all
messed up.

"No, I'm sorry I woke you up."

"Well, I'm sorry that you're down here all alone."

"Well I know, but it's not your job to keep me company. I
won't call you until eight o'clock or so from now on, okay?"

"No, no. Wake me up any time." He yawned and we both
laughed.

Tom was really great. If he saw me struggling with something I couldn't reach, or writing when my hand had gotten
tired and my words were beginning to look like scrambled
eggs, he would say something like "Do you need a hand?

You look like you're getting tired." Sometimes I accepted the help and other times I preferred to struggle. He was fine with both.

Sometimes I would help him too by keeping him company. Once when I was helping him work on his car, he forgot to get the screwdriver out of the tool box. From under the car he called, "Connie, could you hand me that screwdriver?"

"No, you're too lazy," I jested. "Get it yourself."

He treated me like I had a right to exist, a right to have needs and responsibilities like anyone else. Tom also provided me with the means to do things that other able-bodied peers did; he was ingenious in thinking up devices and ways for me to be more comfortable and be able to compete in an inaccessible environment. I was happy just being around him. Tom wasn't in love with me, nor I with him, but we were attracted to each other and talked about it openly.

One of my best friends in college was named Cheryl. One rainy day while we were eating breakfast in the cafeteria, she said smugly, "You don't want to go to class."

"Just because you have a break and you want me to hang out with you doesn't mean I can skip class."

"Yeah, but you don't want to go to class."

"Well no, but that's irrelevant, I have to go to class."

"Why do you have to go to class? You can cut class."

"I can't cut class!"

She pressed, "Why not?"

"I don't know. I never cut a class."

She smiled. "Well, isn't it about time you started?"

So I cut class. It was the longest hour I ever spent. It was great, because the hour felt like it was all mine. I had stolen it from somebody, and now it was mine. We walked around the campus and talked. I loved it. It was the first time in my life that nobody in my family knew what I was doing. I saw the teacher afterwards, and thought "Oh, my god." But he just said "Hi" like nothing had happened.

In high school, and when I had gone to camp, there had been a little of that privacy, but the teachers, counselors and volunteers often told the drivers about the kids' day and the drivers often told the parents. Real privacy was a new-found freedom.

While at Hofstra, I met a student named Charlie. He invited me to go to Bible study with him. He was gorgeous. I had a crush on him, but I didn't think I stood a chance. We went out together as friends, but we never did anything except hold hands. I joined Uncle Gus' Bible Student's Church. Charlie came with me to my church and I went with him to his. Charlie was not prejudiced about disability, so it hurt when he said he would not take me out because I was white. My parents worried about my seeing Charlie. It was all right with them if he was just a friend, but once I mentioned how cute I thought he was, they got really upset. At that point I was relieved that Charlie wasn't interested in me because I didn't know how I could have handled it. I couldn't possibly have snuck around since my parents knew practically everything I did. I remembered Mom finding Glenn asleep with me in my bed back in high school and not freaking out. If she had found me in bed with Charlie like that there would have been hell to pay. I began to wish I could leave home.

I considered the possibility of moving into the campus dormitories. I thought perhaps I could have a roommate help take care of me. I figured OVR might be willing to pay for the dorm instead of transportation. I found out that since I was in a wheelchair and could not walk down the steps independently, I was not allowed to live in the dorms because I was considered a "fire hazard." This made me angry enough that I decided to try to organize people about issues of disability.

I reserved a room and put up flyers saying "Are you a fire hazard? Hofstra University says that disabled students are

fire hazards and cannot live in the dorms. If you are concerned about this issue, please come to a meeting . . ." The
flyer gave a date and time. Five people came to the meeting.
Jimmy, my friend who had joined SDS, was one of them. He
had recently transferred from the community college. We
established a campus organization called People United in
Support of the Handicapped (PUSH). A year later we had
over one hundred and fifty members, including students,
staff, teachers and administrators, with disabilities and without. A number of the members were disabled veterans from
Vietnam. It was important to me that this organization be
inclusive unlike the young adult group I belonged to. It was
important because I had begun to realize that disability oppression, the discrimination based on what someone thinks
another can or cannot do, was not just a disability issue, but
affected all persons. After all, anyone could become disabled
at any moment in their life and even able-bodied people had
varying degrees of ability.

Each year we had Republican and Democratic candidates
for office speak to us about what they were going to do for
their disabled constituency. We offered peer counseling, especially to new students. We made sure we were represented at every campus activity, including campus strikes
and anti-war demonstrations, so as to increase our visibility.

At the yearly carnival, we ran a booth and sold Italian
zeppolis. We bought pizza dough and borrowed electric
frying pans. Cheryl picked up sixty pounds of dough and
put it in the back of her Rambler. By the time she got to
campus and drove through the carnival crowds in the hot
sun, the dough had doubled in size inside her car. It was
quite a sight to see several people in wheelchairs and on
crutches pulling pieces of the dough out of the car. When
we got the dough out, we formed an assembly line to make
the zeppolis. We separated pieces of dough and dropped
them in boiling oil and then rolled them in powdered sugar.
For many of the members of PUSH, this was the first oppor-

tunity they had ever had to interact with the general public. We had a microphone set up and we were hawking these zeppolis. "If you don't know what a zeppoli is you're not hip." Zeppolis became a hit and we made money selling them every year.

Eventually we officially represented the disabled student body to the administration. For instance, if I saw a crack in the sidewalk which might impede a wheelchair user, I would call maintenance and they would deal with it within twenty-four hours. We pushed the administration to make the campus more accessible. We lobbied in Washington, and represented disabled students at the President's Committee for Employment of the Handicapped. We sang Christmas carols at nursing homes and hospitals, and worked with disabled kids so as to reach the disabled population that wasn't in college. We added more and more programs. We started a men's wheelchair basketball team. Some of the women who came to watch became the cheerleaders for the team. We challenged the Harlem Globetrotters to come play us in chairs and it was televised.

After one of our Friday night games, we went to a new local pizza place. The thirty-some odd of us could not all fit in the front area to wait for a table, so about half of us crowded around outside the door. Half were in wheelchairs, a quarter of us used crutches and the other quarter were mainly able-bodied. People inside and outside of the restaurant were staring at us.

"Uh, how can I help you?" a waiter asked.

"Well, we need a bunch of tables and pizzas for thirty people," replied Mark, the team's youngest member. Mark smiled. The waiter frowned and disappeared.

Just then, John, a tall player on crutches, spotted a group of eight patrons getting up to leave. "Let's take the table over there for starters, gang." He began swinging himself across the room towards the table, singing, "Look at us we're walking, look at us we're talking, we who've never walked or talked like this before . . ." It was the theme from the Cerebral Palsy Telethon. Then he changed the words to "Look at us we're walking, look at us we're fucking," and sang at the top of his lungs. The rest of the team joined in.

People were staring, pointing and mumbling. Many got up and left. We filed in and sat around the tables which we pushed together. The waiter came over, still frowning, and asked if we'd like to order.

Mark replied, "Yes sir. Now that there's room for us we'd like thirty cokes and six pizzas. Thank you." The waiter smiled.

We stayed until the place closed. Mark gave the waiter a very large tip and we left laughing and singing. It took a long time to get loaded into the cars because there were no passersby at that time of night who could help. It took three of the paraplegic guys pushing and pulling from different angles to get me into the car.

In addition to my activities with PUSH and my studies, I applied to join the sorority, Kappa Omicron. The sorority sisters were wonderful to me. They lifted me in and out of their cars and drove me to parties. They solicited strong people to carry me in my wheelchair up and down stairs to attend meetings. On "Hell Night" they blindfolded me and switched me around to three different cars just like they did with the other applicants. They thought I was great for going along with them and being so brave and trusting, and I thought they were great for the same reasons. They didn't seem to be afraid of my inability to walk or move very much. They liked me for who I was.

Although I was active and doing well in school, socializing with friends, and changing the world around me, life was far from smooth. I was fast becoming an adult and it was difficult to figure out how or if I could become a wife, mother or working woman and still be disabled. I wanted and needed more control in my life. Mom was too busy to wash my hair more than once a week, and it was always greasy. I felt self-conscious about that, about not being able to fit my body into more adult-style clothing, and about having a more adult-size body which was more and more difficult to lift. My speech was beginning to slur when I became tired.

Most of the other disabled students at Hofstra could push their own wheelchairs. Most of them had strength in their hands and could use a typewriter. Typing a term paper took days for me. Mom helped some, but mostly I typed them on my electric typewriter with my two index fingers. It took about two hours a page. The footnote numbers were the most difficult because I couldn't turn the knob up a half line. I'd con my little brother into coming in and turning it for me. He'd go back and watch TV and I'd type the number. Then I'd wait a while to give him a break and then I'd call him again, and he'd turn it down so I could continue typing the paper. There was no White-Out then, although there was erasable paper. I tried it but I couldn't erase while the paper was in the typewriter. I got Correct-O-Type which were little pieces of paper that you're supposed to slip in between the typewriter key and the paper. I couldn't reach the paper, so I thumbtacked the Correct-O-Type to a pencil eraser. I'd reach over with the pencil, slip the Correct-O-Type in, and hit the key. Every once in a while the key would hit the pencil. The pencil would go flying up in the air and then I had to call somebody to pick it up.

Since my disability seemed to be what made life most difficult for me, as well as for my family, I often hated it, which meant I often hated myself. Sometimes that frustration grew into anger at my whole self, my very existence. My political activity at those times served two purposes. It provided a place where I could feel good about myself because I worked hard. It also helped to change many of the things that caused my frustration.

I had been asking my parents for an electric wheelchair

for some time. Having more mobility would increase my independence and lower my frustration. My father didn't think I could use one, but six weeks before my college graduation he gave me an electric wheelchair as my graduation present.

"Oh, Dad, it's beautiful!" I exclaimed.

"Well, I hope you can use it. It cost a lot of money," he remarked as he lifted me into the new chair. He put my hand on the joystick and turned the switch on.

I pushed and pulled, huffed and puffed, but all I could get the damn chair to do was turn left. "I can't do it, I can't do it!" I cried. My hand went limp as I hung my head and sobbed into my chest. I had failed. My body had failed. I didn't want it, or the chair, anymore.

"I knew you couldn't do it." He threw his hands up in the air. "You wanted it. Now you can't use it. Your mother and I thought maybe you could. I don't know what to do."

Frankie turned on the TV, Dad walked into the other room and I just sat there. I tried to get interested in television. Mom came in announcing, "It's bedtime." She turned off the TV. "Frankie, take your bath now. Pidgie's in bed already, Connie. Are you ready for me to put you in?"

"Yeah," I mumbled, staring off into space.

Mom wheeled me into the bedroom in the new chair. "God, this thing weighs a ton."

The next day at school, I didn't feel like talking to anyone. I barely said two words to Tom while we ate breakfast. On the way to class he asked, "What's the matter?"

"Nothing."

"Why are you so quiet? Don't you feel well?"

I began to cry silently. Tom wheeled me over to a campus bench, sat down beside me and gave me a hug. I sobbed in his arms for awhile. "I . . . I . . . I can't drive my new electric chair. I think my dad is going to send it back."

"Oh, no!" Tom exclaimed. "Don't let him send it back. Listen, it takes babies a long time to learn to walk and it took me about a year to learn to drive a car, so it should take you a long time to learn to use your new chair."

"You think so?"

"Yes, I do. What're you doing Saturday?"

"Nothing."

"Well, why don't I come over and we can practice together?"

"Really? That'd be great!"

That Saturday, Tom and I covered most of Massapequa in that electric chair. By the last hour, I was able to drive pretty well on low speed. Tom was patient and light about my mistakes, even though he was wearing sandals and I inadvertently ran over his feet many times during the day.

Within a few weeks I was whipping around campus and whizzing around shopping malls. As my driving ability increased, so did my depth perception and self-awareness. One time I almost ran into a countertop that was sticking out in the cafeteria. I was yelling, "Stop! Stop!" when I suddenly realized that it was I who had to stop. There was no longer anyone behind me pushing. I gained a remarkable sense of my own power. I raced my other disabled friends down long ramps at the college. I pulled my blind friend, Mickey, around campus on her roller skates. I carried trays of coffee for disabled friends who couldn't push themselves. It was really almost as good as walking.

The day before the ceremony Mom and Dad threw me a big graduation party. I danced in my new chair. There were a hundred people there, including Mrs. Friefeld, my very first teacher. I think she cried more over my graduation than my mother.

The actual graduation ceremony was long but beautiful. It took forever to line up. I was zipping in and out of the line with my electric chair running to-and-fro saying hello to various friends. I couldn't find Tom. Then I saw this guy in a suit that looked like Tom but didn't have a robe on. I started going over to him and stopped. Then I saw Tom right next to him. He caught my eye and came over and said, "Connie, You look great! I want you to meet my brother."

When the commotion died down Tom stood next to me in the procession, and we filed around Hofstra Hall and onto the quadrangle where the ceremony was taking place. People stared as I went by. I sat next to Tom in a row where they had taken out a chair especially for me. As the speaker spoke about our futures and promises and responsibilities, my heart pounded with excitement. I felt ready to take on anything.

10

THE DOG DID IT

After graduation, I had a difficult time. Most of my school friends had left the area, and I had no job. I spent many weeks pursuing help-wanted ads from a newspaper only to find that most of the editing and writing jobs were inaccessible to people in wheelchairs. Those companies that were located in first floor or elevated accessible space had attitudinal prejudices which prevented them from seeing me as an asset to their firm. I sent hundreds of resumes, but was only granted three or four interviews. OVR was no help. Getting rejection after rejection began to hurt more and more.

In order to at least have the opportunity to be out of the house, I volunteered in the Disabled Students' Office at Hofstra. PUSH made me an alumni advisor and a former professor offered me a part-time research position. I spent about half of the week on campus and the other half of the week at home, continuing to look for full-time employment.

One day a very good looking guy in a wheelchair rolled into the Disabled Students' Office. It was a small office, so we sat toe-to toe. We looked at each other and smiled. He said, "Do you know where Dean Seaders' office is?"

"Yes, this is it. Can I help you?" I looked at him closer and added, "You went to Massapequa High, didn't you?"

"Yeah."

"You used to wrestle there."

"Yeah."

I drew in a quick breath and thought, "What the hell is he doing in this chair?" "Recovering," I answered myself.

"I used to watch you wrestle. You're Ron Kovic." My heart started pounding because he was so cute.

He had been wounded in Vietnam. He came in to inquire about starting school at Hofstra the following year. I was still attracted to him, as I had been in high school. We talked for a while. He was still living in the VA hospital, but went home on weekends to his parents' house in Massapequa. We talked about high school and the neighborhood, and laughed about old times. Ron said he'd be discharged soon, and maybe we could get together sometime. He went in to see the dean.

My sister Pidgie was entering adolescence. I hated her. I saw her as greedy. I was jealous of her for being pretty and cute. I couldn't take care of her the way I took care of Frankie because she couldn't physically do things for herself. For instance, when Frankie was little, I taught him how to tie his shoes by verbally directing him. I taught him many things by instructing him. Pidgie couldn't tie her shoes or climb on a chair to reach the sink. She was as badly off as I was. Occasionally Pidgie and I would declare a truce and play a game or watch a show together, but usually at those times it was because she was mad at Frankie and I became her ally. I felt more protective of her when she was little, but as she grew older she became a threat. There was no one in the whole world that was like me. I was unique. I was different, and while that was a problem for some people, the difference also made me special. Pidgie was the only other person in the whole world that looked anything like me. She moved like me, she used the bedpan like me, she was lifted like me, she had to wear the same kind of clothes that fit her contoured body like me and she was brilliant like me. She also was beginning to flirt with my boyfriends, and that pissed me off!

I wanted Pidgie to get the right attitude about herself as a disabled person, even though I usually didn't like her. I talked to her about her rights. I pushed my mother to make sure that my sister was integrated into public school immediately instead of waiting at home for six or seven years as I had to. I encouraged Pidgie to be assertive. I insisted she have an electric wheelchair in grade school so she wouldn't have to struggle as I did, and so she could be more independent. I wanted her to have everything I couldn't have, yet I resented her because she had it. I think she resented me because I was so dependent, and yet I was her big sister. And so, we fought a lot. We were both trying to become adults, and even though we were eleven years apart, we had similar issues because we were still physically dependent on our mother.

It seemed to take my mother forever to get Pidgie ready for bed. I'd be sitting in the living room yawning and waiting for my turn. If my father wasn't home, it seemed to take them even longer. I didn't know why. If I said anything I was told to wait. I felt like an intruder. My mother was very affectionate with my sister, even though she often got angry and hit her. My sister was getting older, and the physical affection my mother showed her upset me. When they sat together, my mother would often hold my sister or stroke her hair. It disgusted me. When I was that age, my mother hadn't held me that way. She held my brother or sister that way because they were little. There were no more babies in the house, but my sister continued to be the baby even though she was an adolescent. I didn't want my mother to hold me that way. I caught myself giving my sister dirty looks when my mother was being affectionate with her. The boundaries between my mother and myself became more blurred and more complex ever since the addition of my sister.

My parents took the family on many day trips. Pidgie enjoyed them a lot, Frankie some, but I hated them. I wanted to be home alone with a friend or going out on my own.

"Let's go for a drive upstate." Dad came through the den jangling his keys and zipping up his jacket.

"Well, I'm going to call Linda and see if she'll come over and watch a movie with me." I picked up the receiver of the phone that was sitting on my laptray.

"No you don't. You're coming with us." Dad took the receiver out of my hand and put the phone on the end table.

"I don't want to go."

Pidgie reprimanded, "Oh, you're so ungrateful Connie. Mommy and Daddy want you to come."

"Why should I be grateful? If they wanted you to go some place you didn't want to go, you wouldn't just go along."

Pidgie stuck out her tongue at me. "You think you're such a big shot."

"You're just jealous!"

I tried hard to be a good older sister to her, but it was hard because we were both so physically similar in our helplessness. Sometimes, when I was struggling for autonomy and adulthood, Pidgie was understanding and even encouraging. Other times she seemed angry at me for no reason that would appear to concern her except perhaps that I reflected her own future reality.

My brother was entering high school. Sometimes I was his pal, but sometimes I was his other mother. One night, when he came home from a party, he was supposed to relieve the babysitter that was watching my sister and helping me. But he came home late and drunk. His friends all wanted to go out on one of their boats in the middle of the night. He was too sick from drinking to go. When they left, he went upstairs to throw up in the bathroom. I called his friends' parents to tell them the kids were out drinking and driving speed boats. Frankie got furious at me for doing that and wouldn't speak to me for weeks.

A couple of months later, one of Frankie's drinking buddies got killed riding drunk in a boat. He fell overboard and got cut in half by the propellers. Frankie was devastated. He grieved privately for several days. One night he came into the den where I was reading and cleared his throat. "I'm sorry."

"I'm sorry about your losing your friend, Frank," I said softly.

"Yeah, I mean I was pretty pissed at you when you told on my friends, but now I know why you did that. Now I understand."

One Saturday morning shortly thereafter, Frankie and I were having a silent late breakfast. We were too tired to talk because both of us had been out late the night before with friends. In the center of the table was a brandy snifter with a goldfish in it. I was staring at it blankly while chewing my toast. The fish tilted from side to side in the water, drifted down to the bottom, and floated up again slowly. I looked up as Frankie was sipping his orange juice. He had been staring at the fish too. Our eyes met.

"I'd give it ten minutes," I said quietly.

"Five."

Pidgie came into the room. "Five what? What are you talking about?"

"The fish," Frank said solemnly.

"That's my fish! I won it last night at the St. Rose of Lima Church's Bazaar. Isn't he cute?"

"It's half-dead," I commented.

"Yeah, those things always die," Frankie added.

"What? What do you mean? It's not going to die!" Pidgie wailed.

Frank and I stared hard at the fish. It slowly rolled over and floated belly up to the surface. Frank and I looked at each other and cracked up laughing. Pidgie screamed, "They killed my fish!"

Mom came running in, shouting, "What happened? What'd you do?"

Neither Frankie nor I could answer her. We were laughing and crying at the same time. Pidgie kept screaming at Frankie and me while Mom screamed at all of us. Frankie went up to his room, and I went into my room to read more want-ads.

That evening I went to a wheelchair basketball game. Ron was on the team now, so I took extra time to look casual but gorgeous. Dad dropped me off at the gym in my manual wheelchair with Linda, an able-bodied neighborhood friend who could push me. If I wanted to go out with friends after the game, I couldn't use my electric wheelchair because it wouldn't fold up to fit in their cars. We got there early. Linda walked over to the cafeteria to get some Cokes, and I hung out, watching the guys warm up.

One of the climbing ropes had been left down near my end of the gym. Ron wheeled over to it, locked his brakes and took the rope in his hands. He looked over at me, smiled and winked. I knew he had been a gymnast before his injury, and I knew his Marine-trained upper body was still in good shape, but I couldn't believe he was going to try this. He climbed that rope from his chair! On the way down he almost missed his wheelchair, but managed to land in it with a grin on his face. He proved he could still do it even though he didn't have the use of his legs. He wheeled over to me and squeezed my hand. My eyes brimmed with tears. "Good luck in the game," I said.

That night he drove me home. I loved watching his muscles ripple as he moved the hand control on the car. It was especially exciting when he braked. After we dropped Linda off, we parked outside my parent's house by the canal. He rubbed my neck and shoulders and we talked. All of a sudden he began shaking and sweating and shouting orders at soldiers who were not there. I realized that he was having a flashback.

My heart began pounding. "It's okay, Ronnie, it's okay. You're in Massapequa now." I kept trying to reassure him, but I was also trying to reassure myself. What if he passed out? What if he got violent and thought I was the enemy? I wondered whether I screamed loudly from the car if anyone in the house would hear me.

Ron began sobbing. He leaned over into my lap and cried and cried. "I'm sorry! I'm sorry!"

We held each other close. I kissed his forehead. He kissed my mouth. We began kissing and fondling. He forgot about Vietnam for a while, and I forgot that my father was waiting to come out and lift me out of the car. Then I heard my father's footsteps on the gravel of the road crunching in between his high-pitched whistling. Ron pulled away. I sat up straight and we both smiled at my father through the window of the car.

That night I dreamt that Ron wrote a book. In the dream, I read the book. It started with a poem, and there was a helmet on the cover with big black letters—something about the fourth of July.

When Ron came to visit the next day, I told him about the dream, but I didn't tell him what the book looked like.

"Who, me, write a book? I don't know." He reached down to his calf to feel if his urine bag was secure. "I think that's a long way off." He looked awful.

"How're you feeling today?" I asked.

"Okay. Not so good, really. I got sick last night."

"Oh, is it your kidneys?"

"Yeah." He looked down at the floor. "Well, no, after I dropped you off I went out and got drunk. I can't really drink much. I get sick."

"Tough memories, huh?"

"Yeah." He looked me in the eyes. "No. It's tough, you know, being in a chair. I don't know how to do it. I'm angry, you know. When I get home my mom yells at me because it's late and I'm drunk. She's talks about God and . . . I don't know. It's hard being there."

"Why don't you get an apartment?"

"I don't know, I'm crippled. Aren't I?"

"No, you're not 'crippled', you're handicapped," I told him. "Most of the guys on the team have apartments and some of them are more disabled than you are."

I pushed him for weeks to get his own apartment. Living at his mother's made him feel and act like a child again. His family's grief and their confusion and anger at what happened to him added to his own anger and grief. They all seemed to be taking it out on each other.

Bobo, my poodle, bounded into the room and Ron played with him for a while. Mom came in and offered us sodas, then left us alone. All of a sudden we heard a trickling sound.

Ron looked around under his chair. "Shit!" he exclaimed. "I'll be right back, my duck leaked."

His urine bag had leaked onto the floor and he went to clean up. He came back in a few minutes and we sat on the other side of the room.

Mom came in with the sodas. She noticed the puddle on the floor. "What's the puddle on the floor?"

"The dog did it, Mrs. Panzarino, honest." Ron looked at me pleadingly.

"Yeah, Mom. I think the dog has to go out."

Mom looked at me and I nodded. I knew that she knew what really happened. "That's all right," she said. "I'll clean it up."

When Mom and Dad were less understanding, it hurt, and there were times when their lack of support increased

my difficulties to the point where they became insurmount-
able. My parents' support was inconsistent. Not knowing
when they would be there for me caused me a great deal of
anxiety, and forced me to face many problems alone, but it
also helped me learn how to get along in a non-caring
world.

One particularly hot afternoon at Hofstra, my cab drove
off without me and I called my father to catch a ride home
with him.

"Well, call them back, talk to the dispatcher," he ordered.
"I'm a busy man."

He taught me how to fight for my rights. "You have a
right to work," he snapped when I was rejected by yet another company. He taught me to expect my rights in the
world, but at home when I wanted to watch a different show
on TV, I was told I didn't have any rights because I didn't
pay enough rent.

I was determined to get a real job so I could pay more
rent and demand more respect at home. The research I had
been doing barely covered the cost of transportation to and
from campus. Special wheelchair van companies cost thirty
dollars per hour. I responded to an ad from *Newsday*, the
Long Island paper. They granted me an interview.

"Dad, thanks for taking off time this afternoon to drive
me to the interview."

We stopped for a light and he looked at me in the rear-
view mirror of his VW van. "Are you nervous?"

"A little." I braced myself in my electric wheelchair for the
acceleration as the light turned green.

"Don't be nervous." He turned a corner. "You're smart;
you did well in school and they should hire you."

I relaxed a bit and tried to take in the support he was offering me. About ten minutes later we arrived in the parking
lot of *Newsday*. We sat in the waiting room of the Personnel
Office.

The interviewer came over to us, introduced himself and

asked, "Would you like your father to come in with you?"
He looked at my dad.

Dad nodded, indicating yes, even while I was shaking my
head no.

The interviewer ignored me and told Dad to follow him. I
followed both of them into a small office. The interviewer
gave a brief description of the job duties and then challenged, "If you worked here, how would you use the toilet?"

"I don't know. I doubt I would ever have to use the toilet."

"But what if you had to?" he pressed.

"I never had to go in college during the day. I doubt I
would have to go here, but if I did, I would have to take the
rest of the day off and go home."

"Oh, I see," he said softly. "If you dropped your pencil or
pen, what would you do?"

"I would ask someone to pick it up."

"What if no one was around?"

Dad looked up from the floor. "Yeah, what if no one was
around?" He looked at me for an answer.

"Well, I guess I would have to have extra pens and pencils
on my desk." My voice began to waver.

The interviewer sighed. "I don't think this is an appropriate work place for you. I'm sorry."

"Yeah, Connie. I think he's right." Dad opened the door
and stepped aside to let me out of the office. He turned to
the interviewer and shook hands. "Thank you very much for
your time."

I didn't speak to Dad all the way home. I was afraid I'd
burst into tears.

"Don't be upset," Dad said sweetly, as he drove. "That
wouldn't be a good place for you to work anyway."

I never allowed him into an interview again. I'd leave him
waiting in the car when I had to. I didn't need to see him
confused as to whose side to be on.

· · ·

When the research job ran out, I worked for Dad in his office for about a month as his bill collector. One day at closing time he put me in his van and went to give a few last minute instructions to his men before they locked up the garage. As I waited in the van for Dad to drive home, I noticed a man in a suit come out of the bar. He was staggering and leaned for a while against a parking meter. I felt sorry for him and worried for his life as he weaved across the street dodging traffic. He leaned up against the front of the van and looked in at me.

The next thing I knew he was in the van stroking my hair and squeezing my breasts. The smell of alcohol was strong, and I was frightened. "My father is right over there if you want my father." I pointed by turning my head towards the plumbing shop.

"I ndho wann yer fadda, I wann yoo."

Just then the van door flew open and my father's workman yanked the guy out of the van. The guy told my father and his men that he just wanted to be nice to me. My father recognized him from a job he had done at the Association for Retarded Citizens (ARC). I was so frightened I was unable to speak. They let the man go, and we drove home.

"Some people are pathetic. You think you got problems, and then you see somebody like that. Makes you feel sorry for them." Dad turned the corner into the driveway, and I burst into tears.

We went inside, and I told Mom and Dad what happened. Dad found out the next day that the man had been fired from the ARC because he had molested two of the retarded women. They said they didn't want to put the women through the torment of court since they probably wouldn't be believed because they were retarded, so they just fired him. Dad reported it to the police, but they never found him.

After a few weeks, I got Dad caught up on all his delinquent accounts and there wasn't much else to do, so I took a job doing home telephone soliciting for Chevron credit cards. I was laid off because I wasn't able to get enough accounts. My supervisor said I was too honest.

I filed for unemployment and received thirty dollars per week. The unemployment officer said he would help me find a job. Once in a while I was able to pick up a temporary part-time research job at Hofstra, but they never lasted longer than three weeks. I would go to the library every morning with a list of the topics I was to research. I would ask the reference librarian to pull the material for me from the shelves. While the librarian was gathering the material, I busily pushed all the chairs away from one of the library tables. Then I would ask him to stack the heavy books up, five high, in various piles around the table. I pulled my chair up to the table and wrote notes in my notepad on my laptray. As I finished with each resource book, I would slide it onto the floor, leaving the next one ready for viewing. The library resounded with a loud "Whump!" each time a book hit the floor.

One day that fall, while I was at home reading the want ads, I got a call from Ron's mother. "Ronnie's in the hospital! He broke his leg last night in his apartment doing his stretching exercises. It was horrible. You could see the bone sticking out. He's in the Bronx VA Kingsbridge. Eli and I are going over in a couple of hours to see how he's doing. Do you want us to pick you up?"

"Yes. Oh my God! Yes." I hung up the phone which was sitting on my traytable. "Mom!" I screamed. "Ronnie's in the hospital. I have to go see him. His parents are picking me up in about an hour or so."

The drive to the hospital was long and tense. Mr. Kovic kept trying to make jokes. As we went through the toll booth in the Bronx, he said to the toll machine, "Hi. How are you today? Our son Ronnie is in the hospital again with a broken leg. He was shot in Vietnam a while ago, so it's pretty serious. Well, you take care now. Have a good day." He tipped his hat to the machine as it clicked the coins.

Mrs. Kovic patted my hand. "He'll be okay. He'll be okay, won't he?"

When we got to see Ron, he looked awful. He was pale and subdued. He had a temperature of 106 degrees.

"Well, at least I can't feel any pain. I have a kidney infection, I think. They can't put my leg in a cast because of the spasms, but I'm going to be all right. Mom, Dad, I'm going to be all right."

"You're going to be fine, Ronnie, just fine." His mother stood up taller.

"Yeah, you'll be fine." His father shuffled his feet. "Let's go get some coffee, Pat, and leave these two alone for a while." He winked at Ron and they left.

"Are you scared?"

Ron started to cry. "Don't let them take off my leg, Babe. I don't want to lose my leg. I know it doesn't work, but I like the way it looks, know what I mean? Don't let them take it," he wailed.

"I'm not going to let them take your leg. I'm right here. I'll be here as much as I can. I love you, all of you, and I don't want them taking any parts of you away."

Ron reached out from under the covers and held my hand tightly. "I'm so scared."

"It's okay to be scared. Only fools aren't scared."

"Yeah, it's okay to be scared. I'm going to be fine, aren't I?"

"Yeah, you're going to be fine, you're just scared." I saw a rat run across the corner of the room and out into the hallway. I tried not to flinch and scare Ron.

For the next six months, I went to see Ron once or twice during the middle of the week using my manual wheelchair, catching a ride with his family or friends. Every Saturday I gave Sam, one of the bus drivers who transported us in the

young adult group years ago, my thirty dollar unemployment check. He would pick me up in my electric wheelchair
at nine o'clock in the morning in his wheelchair van and
drive me to the Bronx VA. He would pick me up again at ten
o'clock at night from the hospital and take me home.

All day long I would carry ice water for Ron, get the
nurses' aides to reposition him on time and check his tubing.
There was a pump that was supposed to keep his leg hy-
drated. It was old and didn't work properly. I would insist
that they check it fairly often. The nurses' aides didn't like
me because I interrupted their card games to insist that they
do their job. Sometimes I was afraid of them, but I never let
them know that.

Ron was in and out of delirium from the high fever. He
was afraid the rats would bite parts of his body that he
couldn't feel and he would get infections. Some of the other
men fed the rats by throwing food in the far corners of the
room, to keep them from eating their bodies. The aides demanded extra money to get patients water or change soiled
bed clothes. If a patient refused to give them the appropriate
tip of ten dollars per day, the patient was often punished by
not being fed or repositioned for a whole shift.

"I feel like I'm in prison," he moaned one day. "Why do
they hate me? What did I do to deserve this? I fought for
this country. They have no respect, no respect." He drifted
off again.

I wept by his bedside. I hadn't known there was so much
hate and pain in the world. Our government had valued
Ron's strong body, turned it into a killing machine, and then
when it broke, tossed it into a living graveyard. There were
twisted and broken bodies all around me. If this is how this
country treats its veterans who have become disabled for a
"cause," it's no wonder they treat people like me, who are
disabled for nothing, as nothing.

Sometimes when I talked to the other veterans down by
the candy machine, I got really pissed. Most of them were

physically able to go home, but they were too scared. They
were having flashbacks. One guy nearly killed his wife in
the middle of the night because he thought she was a
Vietcong. The men were beginning to realize that it had all
been one fucking big mistake and were fighting with themselves and each other in their guilt and pain.

The Sunday afternoon before Christmas, while my dad
was setting up the tree, I went to the early evening modern
music folk mass at St. Rose of Lima Catholic Church. I
prayed for Ron during the communion part of the mass. His
leg had been splintering itself with spasms for several
months, and they could not operate to put a metal pin in it
until they cleared up his kidney infection, which was con-
tinuously causing dangerously high fevers. The kidney infection was due to the stress of the broken leg. Ron was allergic to the antibiotics that would fight the infection. He
had lost weight, strength and spirit.

I prayed for his life. I thought about what the ultimate
sacrifice could be in exchange for Ron's life. I decided that
the biggest sacrifice I could make would be to agree never to
see him again. "Dear Jesus, please let Ron live. I'll give him
over to you and never see him again if you just let him live."

Shortly after I got home, the phone rang. It was Ron's
mother. She was sobbing so hard I couldn't understand her.

"What's happening?" I screamed. "Is he dead? What's
wrong?"

"Nothing. He's fine. The doctor said that a few hours ago
they told Ronnie that the infection was going to kill him
and the only thing they could try was to give him massive
doses of a lot of different antibiotics at once to try to knock
the infection out before his allergic reactions took over.
They said they didn't know if it would work. They said it
might kill him. He told them to try it, and it worked! His
temperature is down and they're operating tomorrow morning. He asked for you, Connie. He asked if we could bring
you in with us tomorrow night to see him when he comes

to. We'll pick you up around five. He loves you, you know."

"Okay," I said. I hung up the phone, barely breathing. God was a fast worker. I didn't know what to do. It would be cruel not to go see Ron, yet I couldn't break my promise to God.

The next morning I talked to the Hofstra University chaplain and explained what happened. The chaplain said that my desire and my sincerity were enough of a sacrifice, and that the Lord would have already taken Ron away from me if He thought that I wouldn't keep my part of the bargain. He said that Ron loved me and needed me at the time and I shouldn't deny him.

January and February brought snow, which increased my isolation. I had to give up Bobo, my dog, because my brother became allergic to him. I wanted to give my brother away instead of Bobo, but I didn't say anything about it. I just cried. I was worried about Ron, getting a job, and my future. My mother seemed increasingly exhausted and desperate. I was needing to be turned in bed more often in the night. Since my sister was now an adolescent, my father could no longer bathe or toilet her at all, so all of Pidgie's care and mine fell on Mom. We screamed and cried at each other. Sometimes she hit me, sometimes she didn't and I wanted her to because I thought it would make her feel better.

One day she decided I should have someone take care of me at night. I still had five hundred dollars from my graduation money. She wanted me to use that money up. I wanted to save it for a car and an apartment. If I did pay someone, I wanted them to take care of me during the daytime so I could go places and do things. My mother wanted someone to take care of me at night so she could sleep. I hired a woman for one night. I didn't sleep that night. I cried and acted like a terrified, angry child having a tantrum. I was horribly embarrassed. My mother was smug.

"You're such a baby. You'll never be old enough to leave home. You'll always want me to do everything for you."

I cringed and looked away.

A few weeks later, in March of 1971, my unemployment ran out. The unemployment officer had not been able to find me a job. He suggested I apply for welfare.

Mom took me down to the Department of Social Services. I was interviewed by a man with crutches that I vaguely remembered from Uniondale High School.

"I'm sorry, but if you are able to work, which you obviously are since you have a college degree and just finished receiving unemployment, I'm afraid you are not eligible for either welfare or Medicaid at this time," he said softly.

"So she can't get anything from you? Not even attendant care?" My mother crumpled up the welfare pamphlet and stuck it in her pocket.

"Where's the Personnel Office?" I asked.

"Just down the hall on your right," he directed, pointing his finger. He waved a little wave as I backed away from his desk.

I zipped into the Personnel Office and asked for the Personnel Director. Shortly after, a blond-haired, made-up, tall woman in loud high heels appeared, saying in a sing-song voice, "Can I help you?"

"Yes," I stated. "I have a college degree, paid for by the State of New York's Office of Vocational Rehabilitation. I do not have any money, and your department said I am ineligible for welfare because I am able to work. Give me a job here at the Department of Social Services."

II

CIVIL SERVANT

I waited three months for the Department of Social Services to make a decision about whether or not to hire me. I called each morning, and each afternoon I received a return phone call stating that the Department had not been able to reach a decision yet. I began to feel more and more desperate. I called Dr. Howard Lord, president of Hofstra University, and made an appointment to see him.

I drove my electric wheelchair into the reception area for Dr. Lord's office. I was dressed professionally and was trying to calm my anxiety so that I could be as articulate as possible. The receptionist looked up and smiled. "You're Connie Panzarino?"

I nodded and smiled back.

"Dr. Lord will be just a few minutes. May I ask why you wanted to see him today?"

"I'm here to see Dr. Lord because I can't get a job and I have a degree from this university."

"Well, I don't think Dr. Lord is the person for you to see. We have a Personnel Office and a Placement Office here on campus, and . . . ?"

"Excuse me, but I don't think you understand. I have been to the Placement Office here and they don't keep files on what jobs are accessible. They don't seem geared to handle the needs of the disabled students."

"You're right," came a voice from behind me. A man with dark hair stepped around in front of me, smiled and put out his hand. "I'm Dr. Lord. Why don't you follow me into my office?" He shook my hand and I followed him into a beautiful carpeted room with plenty of space for my wheelchair. "So, how can I help you?" he asked, leaning back in his chair.

"Well, I don't know exactly, but I do know that it doesn't make sense for the state Rehabilitation Commission to provide tuition and services to educate people like myself, and for a growing university like Hofstra to provide access and a program for disabled students, if after we're educated we cannot find employment. I'm so desperate I applied for welfare, but was told that because I hold a degree I'm not eligible. I applied for a position with the DSS as a caseworker aide three months ago, and they still have not reached a decision about whether or not to hire me. It has been nearly two years since my graduation and I have yet to find a full-time permanent job."

"I admire you, and you're right, although I'm not sure what all we can do for the disabled students right now. I would like to suggest that you speak to your assemblyman, Joe Margiotta. He and I and Jimmy Shuart, Commissioner of Social Services, used to be on the same football team right here on this campus. I'll give Jim and Joe a call, but you call Joe yourself and let him hear it straight from you, all right?"

"Okay. Thank you," I said, puzzled. It all seemed so amazingly simple.

That afternoon I spoke with Assemblyman Margiotta, who agreed to call Commissioner Shuart. The next day, Social Services called me and said I was supposed to report to work the following week.

"See, what'd I tell you, Connie? It's who you know, not what you know," my father beamed, patting my shoulder. "Congratulations!"

None of the supervisors wanted a worker as severely disabled as myself in their unit except Elizabeth Friedman. Her father had been a doctor in the early 1900s and she had an awareness of disability that went beyond that of most of the other supervisors. Her unit was responsible for Medicaid re-certification. My duties on her unit included telephone and face-to-face interviews, financial determination, and recertification of clients.

I started work at Social Services on July 3, 1971. When I got to the office I was delighted to find that my chair could fit under my desk. My phone, though, was another matter. I had asked the Office of Vocational Rehabilitation to provide an intercom phone for me, but they said that since I was working, my case was closed. So I bought a little intercom device for fifteen dollars so I wouldn't have to pick up the receiver, and I rigged it up with a plastic spoon handle and string. It enabled me to answer the phone and dial calls myself. The dialing was quite laborious, but I managed. I hated numbers that had a lot of eights, nines and zeros in them, because those numbers were the furthest away and so they were the hardest to push.

The clerk in our unit agreed to pull my folders from the file for me. She also did considerate things such as unstapling papers and paperclipping them to my folders so I could separate them myself. If I put all the correspondence on top of the folder, she would put it in envelopes for me and mail it all. Another worker that I sat next to was willing to get me the forms I needed for the day. Other workers helped me a lot, and I learned to help them also; I was good at interviewing and liked it, so I did interviews for some of the workers who disliked doing them. It was just like going to school where some of the students had helped me with physical needs and I reciprocated by helping them with their studies. Everyone in the unit worked together. I was continuing to learn to value interdependence over both dependence and independence. There was only one woman in the unit who didn't like me. She was adamant that I should not be taking the space of another person who needed a job when I could collect disability. I tried talking to her about it, but she wouldn't speak to me.

The first few weeks that I worked, I paid for transportation. I took home a hundred and twenty dollars per week. Special transportation cost me ninety dollars per week. The remaining thirty dollars was not enough to live on, even at my mother's. So I decided to buy a car, even though I couldn't drive. I bought a Checker cab and figured out how to put a ramp into it so I could drive my wheelchair up onto it. I put an ad in the paper asking for a driver in exchange for use of my car. I paid for gas and gave the driver ten dollars per week plus use of my car to go to and from their job. I was able to get drivers this way, and the car was available to me after work to go places with my friends.

When I bought the car, my mother withdrew and hardly talked to me for several days. She seemed angry. It became increasingly difficult and confusing to live at home. I had a good deal of responsibility during the day at work, yet after five o'clock and on weekends I was totally dependent on my mother. There were more and more conflicts about family outings. Once I got a job, I thought that meant I would be a full adult with all the rights and responsibilities that went with that. The reality was that nothing had changed. I was still as physically dependent on my family as when I had been six months old, except that now I could talk and pay rent.

I didn't know how to live with the restrictions that I had—the financial limitations, and not knowing if I could ever live on my own, what would happen if something happened to my parents, or how to live in my parents' house where they controlled everything. I had no privacy to be alone with friends, except in my bedroom—but guys weren't allowed in my bedroom. There was so much in my life that I had no control of. I began to experience a strange phenomenon. Some movement of a person's arm, or sound of a voice or a distant car, would trigger a series of visual cartoons, words and sounds as if I were dreaming, but I was awake. They only lasted a few seconds, but they terrified me. I didn't want anyone to know. Without my parents knowing, I started seeing a therapist to try to make sense of my feelings.

I didn't want my mother taking care of me at all anymore, yet I was afraid of having someone else do it. I thought back to Carol, the housekeeper. I had trusted her, but when she had left it had hurt so much. Some of my friends helped me and I tried hiring students on a part-time, short term basis, but even though my mother said she wanted me to have attendants and be independent, she didn't seem to like the people I chose to be my helpers. I was afraid that even if I could hire someone, my mother might get mad at them and they would have to leave, or she might get mad at me and not speak to me, like when I bought my car. Hiring an attendant seemed like betraying my mother's trust, yet not hiring one seemed abusive to her because she had to work so hard. I didn't have enough money to hire a full–time attendant, and my parents said they couldn't afford it either, so my mother remained my full-time caregiver.

Sometimes I felt that if my mother couldn't take care of me, then I was better off dead. I thought about Priscilla, my twenty-five-year-old friend from the young adult group, whose parents were too old to care for her. She lived in a nursing home in my town. I went to see her one night every week right from work and together we would read the Bible and some of the study materials I had gotten from Uncle Gus. I could taste the smell of urine as soon as I came in the front door of her building. I knew I would rather die than end up living in a place like that.

I saw myself as the enemy, the main burden that took my mother away from my father and brother, and made her hit my sister. I had stopped having what my therapist termed hallucinations. I needed to sleep a lot more and give my dream life enough time for my thoughts and feelings to work themselves out. I had been suffering from insomnia and waking up with palpitations and panic attacks. The stress of my not sleeping added to my mother's stress of not sleeping because she had to wake up and deal with me or re-position me. My mother would comfort me and try to calm me down, yet I knew that her anger and frustrations were part of my problem. I felt trapped and crazy every night and on weekends, even though I was a functioning, responsible adult at work each day.

My alarm went off at 7:15 A.M. to wake me for work. "Mom," I called. "I have to get up now."

She was in the kitchen making coffee for herself and my dad. She flipped on the light, walked over to me, and started to turn me on to my back. "You're disgusting!" she exclaimed, recoiling her wet hand quickly from under my mucus soaked pillow and wiping it with tissues. She roughly wiped my face and the pillow, then turned it over. "You're disgusting. No one else would do this. You don't appreciate me."

I thought about the work sitting on my desk at the office. I thought about riding in my car. I thought about my grandmother holding me when I was little. It was too painful to be present in my body with her, so I let her move it and wash it and dress it and put it in my wheelchair. I would catch up with it later, after it left the house.

After two years working in Medicaid recertification, I was transferred to Medical intake, where I did all the initial interviewing and screening with a man named Henry. Henry had been the person with a disability who had first interviewed me when I applied for financial assistance.

I began to realize that the Medicaid rules worked against people who needed it. The rules were made to appear as though we were helping people, but we didn't help people get free of the poverty, racism or disabling conditions that made them need medical assistance in the first place. Medicaid paid for major illnesses, but it wouldn't pay for vitamins to keep somebody healthy.

When abortion was covered for the first time under Medicaid, many women saw this as a victory. What they did not realize was that there had also been cutbacks in monies available for women who wanted to keep their children. The state agreed to fund abortion only because they realized that if they paid for abortion, they wouldn't have to pay to support as many children. When pregnant women came into Social Services for financial medical assistance, they were immediately directed to my office and told to apply for a Medicaid-funded abortion. Women thought that was their only option. I broke rules by telling them they didn't have to have abortions, that they could have their child and receive welfare payments for medical and living expenses. I was not against abortion; I was pro-choice.

At first, my job at Social Services made me feel important because I was a civil servant. But the longer I stayed there, the more radical I became. From my family's perspective, too many Medicaid and welfare payments were being given to people who didn't need them. My parents and their friends told me that people on welfare and Medicaid were driving Cadillacs and living off of the backs of the hard-working middle class. Jimmy and Ron, though, were telling me the opposite, and what I saw at DSS proved to me that they were right. I learned very quickly that welfare standards were way below what anybody could live on—a family of four in 1973 was expected to live on less than four hundred dollars per month. Some of the other DSS workers taught me how to make math errors to help qualify people who really needed services.

In order to save money during campaign time to make a certain politician look good, the Commissioners would suddenly hand down new policies which would affect large numbers of recipients. For instance, on a Monday morning we might get a notice that from ten o'clock in the morning until one o'clock in the afternoon, any recipient between the ages of sixty-eight and seventy-two in the north part of Long Island should have their case closed. It was a tremendous amount of work to close so many cases, and the policies were surely illegal, but the result was that the number of people on the welfare rolls would go down for that week. It wouldn't matter that when the people got their letters at the end of the week all they had to do was ask for a fair hearing, and a month or two later when they won their hearing, their medical bills would be covered even for the time they were cut off. Some people didn't know they had been cut off illegally, so they never reapplied. I often wondered what happened to them.

While the county and state officials were manipulating the Social Service offices, the state and federal governments were busy manipulating student activism on college campuses. The colleges built rathskellers and bars, and sponsored wine and cheese parties on campuses. The recreation funding for campus organizations increased dramatically. There was a lot more drinking. Drugs were being sold much more openly and in greater quantities than when I had been a student. Young students, even the disabled ones, became more concerned with the hours the campus bars were open than they were with the role their colleges took in national civil rights issues. PUSH's membership dwindled as disabled students became more concerned with fitting in at parties than with fighting for access to class. When students were too drunk or stoned to get angry, there were far fewer demonstrations. There were still clear angry voices in the struggle, but we were becoming few and far between.

Ron and I spoke to or saw each other at least twice a week. We strategized as he began speaking in high schools all across the country. His hope was that the young boys he spoke to would never want to go into the service. Sometimes he would go and hang around outside the recruiting stations and try to talk with boys before they went in. He told them how the recruiters would lie to them, as they had lied to him, about benefits, pay, safety and patriotism. He was driven to make sure that what happened to him didn't happen to anyone else. Ron would show the kids his leg-bag and his scars, and tell them about the rats in the veterans' hospitals. He talked to them about love of all people, as opposed to the patriotism that had made him kill Vietnamese babies.

Ron began organizing disabled veterans across the country. As he did, my political world was broadened. I realized more and more that it wasn't just local officials, local libraries and school districts that needed change. Oppression was much more widespread than that. I started thinking more about my parents, passively supporting leaders and a lifestyle that oppressed a lot of other people. Their generation was taught not to question the rules. They believed that that would make them safe. I was quickly learning that the rules weren't made for non-white people, poor people, or people like me.

Although I was doing much better in therapy, I continued to wake up at night with my heart pounding. On several occasions it occurred during the day, and I was frightened that that meant that I was going to begin having hallucinations again. I was afraid to tell our family doctor, because I thought he might put me on tranquilizers. Being on tranquilizers meant being dependent on drugs. It would make me feel like a drug addict. When I finally told him, he did some cardiology tests. It turned out that I had a condition called tachycardia. I was put on medication for it, and within several weeks was able to sleep at night. I was still having a good deal of anger and anxiety, but without the physical palpitations I was able to function more clearly. It was also a relief to my mother not to have to get up and down in the middle of the night. It was wonderful to know that I was not going to be crazy; being disabled was enough.

My sister Pidgie, who now was wanting to be called Patricia, and I began to become friends. She had also been afraid that I was becoming crazy, and had not wanted to talk about it. I guess she felt like whatever happened to me was going to happen to her.

One night I was sitting in the den embroidering while my father was watching the news coverage of the 1972 Republican National Convention. All of a sudden there was a great commotion as three disabled veterans disrupted the Convention. There was Ron, sitting up on the armrest of his chair, as tall as he could be, shouting out about the injustices of a war that wasn't a war and about how the American people were being lied to and its young boys crucified. I cried as the police dragged him off. I was proud of and afraid for him.

"Son of a bitch! Look at what a disgrace he is to this country. He'd better not come around here anymore. If you know what's good for you, you won't even talk to him. If Assemblyman Margiotta ever knew you hung out with people like *him*," my father nodded toward the TV, "he wouldn't have helped you get a job. He'd probably even get you fired."

I knew right then that I had to find a way to live on my own. I was not giving up Ron, or my beliefs.

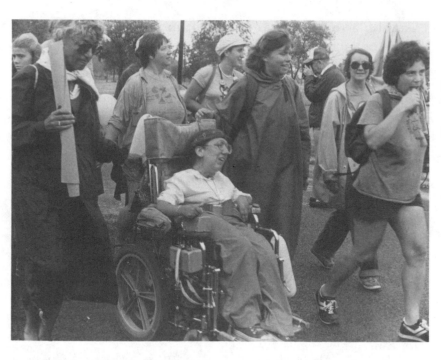

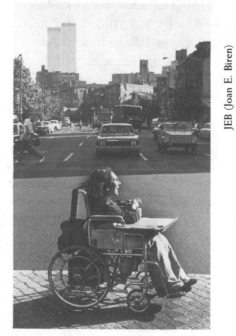

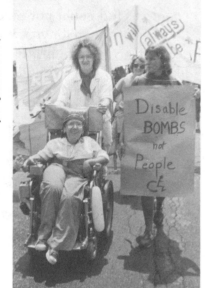

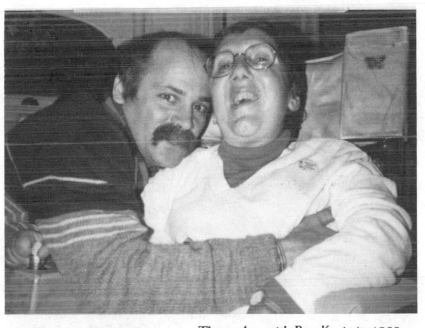

Judy Brewer

The author with Ron Kovic in 1989.

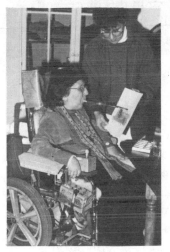

Nancy A. Clover

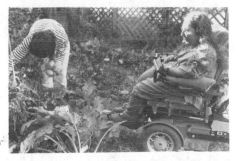

Chiselle McGee

12

THE GREAT ESCAPE

"Priscilla, we're moving," I announced triumphantly at our weekly visit at the nursing home.

"Connie, what are you talking about?" She looked at me as though I were crazy.

"I'm taking off next Monday and going to look for an apartment for us. I'm sick of seeing you live in this place, and I'm sick of living where I can't be myself. My parents won't let Ron come to the house anymore, so how am I supposed to see him?"

"How're we going to do it?"

"The minute you move out of this dump, you'll have your SSI and SSDI checks to help pay rent. We can split the rent, and I'll pay all the utilities because I'm working. You can get an attendant through Medicaid and I'll pay for her food and other expenses. We can give her a free place to live and she can take care of both of us. The Bible students said they would help us build a ramp and get furniture."

"Really?" Her eyes filled up with tears.

"Of course! You just keep praying about it, keep your fingers crossed and have a little faith in me."

"You know you're going to have to sign a paper that says you're willing to take full responsibility for me, don't you?" Priscilla looked at me seriously.

"Yeah, so what? I'd rather be responsible for you than let

you die in this hole." I blinked back angry tears, took a deep breath and sighed. "By the way, I forgot to tell you, I've decided to get baptized Sunday. Uncle Gus is going to do it in Brother Ed's pool."

I had been studying more frequently with the Bible students who were introduced to me by my Uncle Gus. All the Bible stories and pamphlets he had sent to me when I was growing up had an important impact on my spirituality. The Bible students were progressive pacifists who believed that there was no hell and that God had made beautiful promises to everyone, even those who didn't believe in him.

The Sunday night that I was baptized, I prayed hard that God would help me find an apartment. I found an apartment on Monday. By Tuesday I had hired a live-in aide from a housekeeping agency. All my prayers had been answered. I was almost free. I thought about Charlotte, my therapist, who was away for the summer. Would she ever be surprised when I sent her my new address and phone number.

When I showed my parents the lease, my mother remarked, "Well, so you have an apartment, when are you moving?"

I replied, "Well, probably by the weekend."

"Well, why not sooner?" she asked. "Why do you have to wait so long if you have the apartment now?"

I was stunned.

I had the new attendant, Jean, work for me at home for a few days so that I could train her and she could help me pack. She had been brought up in a convent in Antigua. During the interview, she told me she would never get married. She said she was going to be a virgin and devote herself to God and taking care of disabled people. This was apparently what she thought she had to say to get the job. Once she realized I was a regular person, she dropped the facade and admitted that she had about six boyfriends and a daughter in Antigua. We got along great.

When I called the Bible students to tell them Priscilla and

I were moving, they called each other and rounded up beds, linens, a kitchen table and chairs for us. I'd already been saving free glasses from the gas station. I went to Woolworth's to buy cheap dishes and silverware. We moved all of my stuff in on Thursday, and on Friday I went to sign Priscilla out of the nursing home. It felt great to get her out. I felt like hiring a band. The nursing home staff thought we were crazy, but they did release her and her belongings to me. If they hadn't, we would have snuck her out. Jean drove my Checker cab. Priscilla and I just fit in, knee-to-knee, with her stuff piled all around us. It was a maroon Checker cab with a black vinyl top. We called it our getaway car. We got to the apartment, unloaded everything, and then took Priscilla down to my office at Social Services where she applied for and received attendant care through Medicaid.

Living in the apartment was exciting and challenging. My brother and sister loved it because it gave them a place to hang out. When my parents came to visit they decided I needed a couch, so they bought me one. When Charlotte, my therapist, came back, she was so proud of me she hugged and kissed me. She also helped us out by giving us a couple of dressers and a nice set of dishes.

I suffered from anxiety much of the time. It was actually less than when I lived at my parents' home, but it was still present. Mostly I just rode out the fear, like a wild horse bucking underneath me, threatening to throw me off into outer space. It was as if all the terror and pain of my childhood was coming up now that I was in a safe place. I tried to ignore it when I could, and when I couldn't, I called Charlotte. She was always there for me and never got angry, even when I called her several times a day.

I worked at DSS, while Priscilla supervised the housekeeping and cooking. Weeknights we watched TV, or sometimes the Bible students came over for Bible study.

Sometimes Priscilla and Jean would go to Bingo while I went to campus events. On weekends we went to bars. I noticed that if I sat with a cigarette in my hand and a beer in front of me, people talked to me, and if I sat with a Coke, they treated me like a social outcast. After a while I realized I didn't have to ruin my body by smoking or drinking. I could just live my life doing what I wanted and be happy. I soon found myself making friends with others who felt the same way. Being happy with my disability became my declaration of total rebellion against what society expected and what my family had prepared me for.

I went through a second adolescence at twenty-three. Once I even hid from Jean behind a car in a parking lot for a long, long time. I had never been able to run away as a child. She searched for me for almost an hour and then gave up. I finally came back on my own. We didn't talk about it; I think she understood.

It was very hard to get aides to relieve Jean on weekends because few women wanted to take care of two disabled individuals for seventy dollars a weekend. Sometimes my friend Kathy and my blind friend Mickey came to take care of both of us. They agreed to work over Labor Day weekend, split the money between them and spend time hanging out with us. On Labor Day, we ran out of clean washcloths and towels. I insisted we had to do the laundry.

It was over ninety degrees out, and I had my period. Since it was so hot, I was wearing a little smock shirt. I didn't have shorts on under it, just a pair of underpants with my Modess pad. Mickey said she knew what it was like to not have any clean towels or washcloths, so she agreed to help me do the laundry while Kathy stayed home with Priscilla. Mickey said we could walk the three blocks to the laundromat if I went ahead of her in my electric wheelchair. She would follow the sound of my chair while pulling the laundry cart behind her. I had a bit of difficulty steering the chair because it was so hot my hands were sweating, and the heat also made me more fatigued. The heat made it hard to breathe or move, and my menstrual cramps were making my head spin.

Just opposite the laundromat on Clinton Street, the bumpy sidewalk pitched me abruptly towards the street. I lost control of the chair. I knew I was going to go over the curb. I tried to aim for a telephone pole to break my fall, but missed. So I hit the joystick as hard as I could, praying that I could hop the curb. Instead, I landed upside down in the street, entangled in my chair, with a car coming directly at me. Mickey was yelling, "Where'd you go? Where are you? What happened?"

I shouted, "Mickey, quick, wave your arms. There's a car coming at me!"

She waved her arms wildly and the car screeched to a halt. A man and woman jumped out and ran over to me. They started trying to disentangle me from the chair. "Oh my God!"

"Jesus Christ!"

"Who's responsible for this?"

The man directed Mickey, "Grab her foot, move her arm."

Mickey was confused since she couldn't see what was happening. "Leave her alone," I moaned. "She's blind."

A woman shouted, "Who is responsible for these people being out here alone?"

A passersby, by this time, had run up to the scene and somehow gotten me back into the wheelchair. I was sitting at such an angle that my right hip was partly on the armrest of my chair. My smock had gotten so twisted and bunched up that my hip and butt were uncovered. Somebody ran to call an ambulance.

I said, "I don't want an ambulance. Please call my uncle at 485-3683 or Dr. Madonia at 741-6222." I knew that my parents were out-of-town for the weekend and I was afraid that if someone saw their names in my wallet, they would try to call and get no answer. I was concerned that if I lost consciousness or lost control, that they might do the wrong thing to me, like lift me incorrectly or give me medication that would add complications to my disability or conflict with medication I was already on. I kept chanting the names and phone numbers over and over.

A policeman came. "Officer, she needs to go to the hospital," said a stout lady in a pink dress.

"I don't want an ambulance. Please call my uncle at 485-3683 or Dr. Madonia at 741-6222."

"Call an ambulance," said the man who had stopped his car.

"I don't think she can walk," said a mother holding her baby.

"I don't want an ambulance. Please call my uncle at 485-3683 or Dr. Madonia at 741-6222."

"The other one can't see," said an old man with a cane.

"They have places for people like that," chortled the lady in the pink dress.

"I don't want an ambulance. Please call my uncle at 485-3683 or Dr. Madonia at 741-6222."

"Officer, she needs a doctor," the mother with the baby insisted.

An old man came over, put a hand on my shoulder and wiped at my eye with a dirty handkerchief. It was full of blood. "Relax, honey. You don't realize it, but you cut your eye and I'm afraid that you need attention for it." I started to get freaked out. Mickey came over and looked in my eye and said, "It's not really that bad. You'll be fine."

I said to myself, "Good. She's blind. She knows about eyes. I'm going to be okay." Then I realized that since she was blind she couldn't see a damned thing. I shouted "Mickey, what do you mean!" Then I turned to the policeman and repeated the names and numbers several more times. When he continued talking to everyone but me, I shouted, "FUCK YOU, YOU SON-OF-A-BITCH! I'm the one who's hurt! I am an adult. Why are you listening to them and not talking to me?" Everyone became very quiet and nervous.

He asked, "What do you want me to do? Do you want an ambulance?"

I said for the hundredth time, "I don't want an ambulance. Please call my uncle at 485-3683 or Dr. Madonia at 741-6222."

"Okay, okay, I'll go call your uncle." He walked across the street to use the pay phone in the laundromat.

Uncle Pete came within five minutes with my cousin, Nick. They strolled over to me from their car, grins on their faces. Uncle Pete said, "Heard you need a ride home." He looked around at the police and crowd, and said jovially, "Why didn't you call sooner? It's almost dinnertime." They lifted me into their car. Mickey offered to push the wheelchair home. When we got home, Uncle Pete put salve on my wounds and checked my eye. It didn't need stitches, I just had a cut in my eyelid. He told me to take my usual medications and go to sleep.

Two hours later there was still no sign of Mickey. My uncle and cousin went out searching the surrounding streets for her. She had gotten disoriented; they found her two miles in the opposite direction.

The next day when Jean came home, she shouted as she came in the front door, "What the hell went on in this house this weekend?"

I asked timidly from the bedroom, "Why?"

"Because I've been pulling your underwear and nightgowns off of bushes and fences from here to Clinton Street, that's why!" In the confusion, Mickey had dropped all the laundry.

That evening, I looked in the mirror. I looked like a prizefighter. I had two black eyes, and scraped up cheekbones. Ron came over that night and we made out for hours. He laughed, saying, "This is like making out with Joe Louis."

The next day I went to work. People were astounded at the way I looked. Someone suggested that I sue the town for bumpy sidewalks. When I asked Mickey if she thought it was a good idea she squawked, "Right! They're really going to believe a blink."

Jean left, having only worked for us for three months. The next two years, Priscilla and I had about eighty different aides. It was a lot to ask of one woman to take care of us both for thirty-five dollars per day, even with room and board. The aides didn't even have their own room. Priscilla, myself and the aide all slept in the same bedroom. When Ron stayed over, or Priscilla had a friend visiting, some of us would stay in the living room on the sofa-bed.

The agency sent us aides whose alcoholic husbands came banging on the door in the middle of the night. They sent us aides who left us alone "for five minutes" to run an errand and didn't come back until hours later. The agency sent us aides who encouraged us to achieve independence, and others who stole money, clothes and food from us. Some of the aides brought us presents, and some aides brought their children to work and beat them in our bedroom. They sent us aides who came in, looked at the two of us, and walked out the door before they even knew our names.

They sent us Hispanic aides, African-American aides, Asian aides, German aides, Italian aides, young aides and old aides. We learned about many different cultures from them. Most of the aides they sent us wouldn't listen to us and wanted to do things their way. A few of the agency aides wanted us to direct them. The agency sent aides who wanted us in bed at seven o'clock as if we were children, and aides who were ill with staph and strep, so we became ill. One of their aides wouldn't let us have hot soup and a cold drink together because we were "invalids," and also believed we had to be washed with cold water. The agency sent us aides who brought guns into our house. We were afraid to ask them to leave, because we couldn't live without them and were afraid of retaliation. Slowly we learned how to hire and train and manage our own attendant care. When we found a good attendant, we would send them to register with the agency so they could be paid by Medicaid.

Eventually we found Fran. She was not the perfect attendant, but she cared about us and set limits for herself. One afternoon I said, "We want chicken tonight, Fran. Okay?"

"Sure."

Three hours later, Priscilla said, "Gee, I really want to go to Burger King."

Fran said, "You mean I cooked all this food and you two want to go to Burger King? What? Are you crazy?"

"Yeah."

Fran said, "Fine, I'll put it in the fridge. We'll have it tomorrow. Let's go to Burger King."

Fran seemed to be very comfortable with her own sexuality and ours. She often encouraged each of us to date and to enjoy our bodies. She encouraged us in areas that no one else ever did. For instance, she was surprised that I had never seen my whole self naked in a mirror, and encouraged me to look. Somehow it felt wrong to look at myself. It took me several weeks before I had the courage to ask her to wheel me in front of the mirror after my bath. I was surprised to see that I was not as deformed as I thought I was. Something changed inside me. I remembered the Connie in the mirror of the credenza. Maybe it was all right if I couldn't walk like her.

The next day, when Ron called from California where he had been spending part of the winter and said he wanted to come over and play Monopoly, I told him I didn't want to play Monopoly anymore. I told him I was tired of playing Monopoly, I wanted to make love with him. He was a little shocked, I think, since I had never been that forward before, but he seemed pleased. He flew home the next day and we spent the night in the Chelsea Hotel.

While Ron took a bath, my attendant, Fran, undressed me and put me into bed. I used the bedpan and then put on my pink nightgown with lace trim. Ron came out of the bathroom, and my attendant left. He had a towel across his lap. We both looked at each other a little shyly. "Alone at last," I said, and we both giggled. Ron shouted, "Close your eyes Panzarino," threw back the covers, jumped into bed and covered himself up as he flung the towel onto the floor.

Ron dimmed the light by the bed and rolled over facing me. He began playing with my hair and touching my face. I stroked his arm and his shoulder. He slipped his arm around me, under my waist and pulled me to him. "Are you sure you don't want to play Monopoly?" he asked.

"I'm sure." We started kissing. He kissed my face, ears, neck. He sucked on my ears. He pressed my face into his chest. He put my hand on his nipple as he fondled mine. I was surprised when he had an orgasm through his breasts. He rubbed my legs and put his hand between them to bring me to orgasm. At first, he wasn't very interested in my touching the parts of his body he couldn't feel a lot, but the closer we got the more he began moving my legs over his. He didn't have any feeling in his penis and it was hooked up to his urinary bag. He didn't use his penis in the lovemaking. I was relieved, because I had never seen a penis and was afraid of intercourse.

We made love for hours. Fran and Priscilla were in another hotel room that Ron paid for, so if I needed to go to the bathroom we could call my attendant on the phone.

"What would your mother say if she knew where you were now, Miss Panzarino?" Ron laughed.

"Knock it off."

He rolled over, kissed me, and we both fell asleep.

A few months later, I went out to California with Kathy, my friend who often took care of me, to visit Ron for two weeks. I went to help him organize for the American Veterans Movement (AVM). From the moment I got off the plane I had no anxiety. I felt far enough away from my parents and family problems to finally feel separate and safe.

I found Ron in a filthy two-room apartment with ten guys. They came there to rest from an encampment for disabled Vietnam veterans. Over one hundred disabled veterans and their supporters had been living outside in tents at a state university for several weeks to protest the mistreatment of Vietnam veterans by the government.

I began to clean up with Kathy. When she went to empty the bedpan in the bathroom, there was a rubber urinary bag floating in the toilet, which was stopped up. Kathy burst into tears. I said, "It's okay, Kathy. Don't worry, we'll deal with it."

"Dan, can you get your duck out of the toilet so we can get it working?" Dan was a paraplegic who, like Ron, had been injured in the war that had still not been declared a war.

"Thanks. Kathy, get a hanger and untwist the wire at the top so we can use it to clear out the toilet stoppage. Peter, help me clear out the toilet stoppage in a couple of minutes."

"I hate shit." Peter was an angry Asian-American veteran with burn scars over his arms and face.

"You'll hate it more if you have to carry yours around all day with no toilet to put it in, so don't give me any grief."

I called and ordered food, and began to answer the phone, giving out media information, directions to the encampment, and organizing volunteers to support the encampment.

"I'm sure glad you're here, Babe." Ron was putting on a tie, in preparation for a talk show, as the other guys were getting into vans to go back to the encampment. When we were alone Ron said, "I can't trust everybody. Watch out for Martin. And don't forget women are agents too. Now that we're organizing nationwide, it's getting more complicated."

"You don't have to tell me. I'm getting so tired of my phone being tapped in New York because of your activism. First I didn't believe you, Ron, when you said that the clicking noises on the phone were phone taps. Remember when you told me you were going to land in Atlanta, that day when I knew you were going to be in Boston, and right after you hung up someone called to asked me what time they should meet your plane in Atlanta? I knew it was phoney information, so I knew someone had to be listening in on us. Oh well, at least if there's a fire, I won't have to dial the fire department. I'll just pick up the phone and ask the FBI to send help. Look, I'll call you once in the beginning of the talk show, to set you up with a leading question, and then I'll do a call-in at the end to add whatever they didn't let you say."

"Great, 'Maria.' Who are you going to be during the second call?"

"Francesca! I'm feeling exotic."

"You look exotic." He grabbed me and kissed me. "How's my tie?"

"Everyone will love it on the radio. Do you want me to comment on it when I call you?"

"Don't you dare." The vans began beeping for Ron. "Gotta go. I'm sending you back five or six guys, but Liz says she'll drop by and give you a hand tonight," Ron said. Liz was one of his other lovers. Ron was not monogamous by nature. Although he and I were in a solid relationship, he had other lovers as well. I had mixed feelings about Ron having other lovers. Sometimes I got mad at him. One night when we were arguing about it, he said he didn't think we should have so many cats. He said we should just have one cat because we couldn't love more than one cat. I smiled and realized that I had the capacity to love many people, many children, and certainly many cats, so maybe he had the capacity to love more than one woman.

"Ross is having a lot of flashbacks, so maybe a good

night's sleep will help him out," Ron added giving me another quick kiss.

We got a lot of media coverage that week. Ron was on about eight radio and several TV talk shows. I was also interviewed several times by the press. I slept little and worked hard. I wound up with bronchitis that week so I went to the local hospital in Long Beach. The emergency room personnel looked at me like "Oh my God, what happened to her?" I said, "Look, I'm always this way, I'm just here 'cause I'm congested, I have a cold. I'm always in a wheelchair. Just give me some medicine and let me get out of here."

On Easter Sunday, Bob, a strong vet who got into using a lot of drugs in Vietnam, and Shannon, his pregnant wife, took us to the encampment to be with Ron and the guys. There were church choirs, media and guys all over the place. And I thought "Wow, what a great way to spend Easter Sunday." We had beer and pretzels for breakfast.

The encampment lasted longer than we expected. Kathy and I flew back to New York. I began to set up speaking engagements and rallies across the country for Ron and several other guys from the AVM.

Soon after I came back, Priscilla decided to move out with Fran. She and Fran had realized how much easier it was without me. I knew they were right because it had been wonderful to have Kathy as an attendant all to myself while I was in California. Sometimes living with Priscilla and an attendant felt like living at home with my sister and my mother, each of us competing for the care we needed. But I didn't know if I could survive alone financially in the apartment without Priscilla. I didn't think I would be eligible for attendant care, since I was employed. I didn't know what I was going to do, but I knew I wasn't going back home.

13

A NIGHT
IN THE CHAIR

Several days before Priscilla left, I filled out a Medicaid application for attendant care services and handed it in at my office. I knew that the application process could take several months, so I advertised in the newspaper for someone to provide attendant care for me in the meantime, in exchange for free room and board.

The first woman I interviewed was an alcoholic. She said she was trying to stop drinking by going to AA meetings, but she still needed several beers a day and a few hard drinks at night. I didn't hire her, but I kept her name and number because she said if I ever needed a ride somewhere she could drive me and would not drink for at least a couple of hours beforehand.

Joan, the first woman I hired for this arrangement, seemed pleasant enough for the first few days. Then one day as a friend of mine was leaving the apartment, Joan picked up a glass bottle and threw it at my friend because she "didn't like her hair." I heard the bottle break on the sidewalk, but couldn't see my friend's reaction. I was scared at the thought of being left alone with this woman.

That afternoon I laid down to take a nap. Joan was supposed to wake me after an hour, but she didn't. When I woke up I could see the clock from my bed, and knew it had been almost two hours.

"Joan!" I called out. "Joan, Joan." No one came in. "Joan! Joan!" I screamed louder and louder. Still no one came. I began sobbing for her. "Joan, please come in. Help! Help! Joan! Are you there? Is anyone there?" I yelled and cried and shouted for nearly an hour. My stomach began to hurt and I became nauseated. I screamed and sobbed, trying to keep my stomach under control. "Help me, somebody! I'm going to throw up!"

Another half hour went by. Joan glided silently into the room and stared at me.

"Where have you been? Haven't you heard me calling you? I was going to throw up. Why didn't you answer me? Why didn't you come in?"

"You're not sick," Joan said with a blank expression.

"How do you know? I could have died in here. If I vomit laying down, I choke. I could have died."

"When it's time to die, we die." She folded her hands on her chest.

My heart began pounding. Just then the phone rang. Joan answered it. She brought the phone and put it by my ear. "Hello," I said. "Who is this?"

"It's me, Babe." It was Ron.

"Ron, I need you to come over now, and bring Kathy, okay?"

"Something's wrong, isn't it? It's that weird attendant. I didn't trust her. It'll be fine. I'll be right over."

Ron came with Kathy and they got me up out of bed. Joan was in the living room walking around in circles, talking to herself. I asked her to leave and Kathy stayed through the weekend.

That Monday I went to work and Kathy went to school. Halfway through the morning the director of medical services, Mr. Rosa, stopped me in the hallway, shouting, "What do you mean by this?" He was waving a Medicaid application in my face. "You know you're not disabled."

I looked down at my wheelchair, then looked up at Mr. Rosa. "Excuse me, sir? What are you talking about?"

"This application of yours for medical assistance for attendant care. You know if you're working you're not disabled. That's the law. I'm going to tear this up."

"No! If you're going to deny me Medicaid, I want it in writing and I'll fight you all the way!"

During my lunch hour that day I called the Office of Vocational Rehabilitation. They said they could not help me. I went down to the welfare office in my building to apply as a worker whose income did not meet her living expenses, since some of those expenses included attendant care. I was denied welfare because if one of my working expenses was attendant care, that meant I was disabled, and the welfare office could not help people who were disabled. They referred me to Social Security.

I went back to my desk to work. Kathy called and said that her mother would not let her help me out during the week because she had to go to school, but she said Ron would be there when I got home. I told my co-workers about my dilemma. Some of them were empathetic. Others thought the laws were justified, otherwise anyone could get disability. A few workers offered to drive me in my car to and from work for a couple of weeks if that would help out, but no one offered to help me go to the bathroom, except a new woman who worked in the records office and had cerebral palsy. She came home with me that afternoon to help me go to the bathroom, she prepared supper and then left me with Ron.

Ron felt bad that he couldn't lift me onto the bed or couch so I could lie down to sleep. I was afraid I would slip and get hurt. That night we vacillated between being upset that he couldn't take care of me, being upset that I couldn't take care of myself and being determined to survive anyway.

"Fuck those able-bodied Watergate assholes in Washington," shouted Ron.

"Yeah! Fuck them. Who are they to say I can't work and still be disabled."

"Fuck them all!" Ron said.

"Yeah! Fuck them all!"

We looked at each other and smiled.

"I'd like to fuck you right now," said Ron.

"I wish you could too."

Ron, knowing I wasn't going to sleep well sitting up in my chair, tried to stay awake with me. We talked for hours. He eventually got too tired and we both fell asleep, my legs on top of his lap on the couch. Making it through that night was our own little rebellion.

That next morning when my friend Allen came to drive me to work I was stiff and sore. I had a dry breakfast in the cafeteria—no liquids because I could not use the bathroom. Henry, in my office, said I looked like hell, so he took most of the intakes for the day and let me just do paperwork. In between working and yawning I called every state and federal representative I could think of to try to get some sort of waiver so I could have attendant care. I called Mickey to see if she had any ideas.

"You what? You spent the night in the chair? Why didn't you call me?"

"I don't know. I feel bad bothering everybody."

"Listen, it's going to take you at least a week or two to resolve all this. Why don't I pack my bags and meet you at home? I can give you two weeks of personal care. What are friends for?"

I started to cry. For the first time in two days I would get a whole night's sleep, and be able to go to the bathroom when I needed to. Several friends had suggested I go back home to live with my folks, but I just couldn't do that. They weren't getting any younger and neither was I.

• • •

I took the next day off and went to Social Security with Mickey. Ron's mother gave us a ride. I applied for Supplemental Security Income (SSI) because that would give me automatic Medicaid benefits to pay for attendant care. I filled out all the forms, reading them all to Mickey to share them with her as I completed them. When my turn came, I led Mickey in with me. The man behind the desk read my application and laughed. "What is this, a joke? You're not disabled. You're working full time at DSS!"

"What are you, blind?" screamed Mickey. "Can't you see she's in a chair?" she said, rapping his desk with her white cane.

"Mickey, stop it! Excuse me, sir, but if I'm not eligible may I have a letter in writing so that I can appeal the decision?" I tried to remain calm while Mickey began cursing and swearing.

"Connie, don't let these assholes screw you over. Quit your job and go on disability. You have to have attendant care or you're going to die."

The man at the desk cleared his throat. "I'm sorry but since we know that you're *able* to work, we would have to deny you benefits even if you quit your job."

Mickey turned very red in the face. I zipped out the door shouting, "Let's go, Mickey." I did not want to have her arrested on my account.

The next day I called the Secretary of Health, Education and Welfare, Caspar Weinberger, in Washington, D.C. After being transferred seven or eight times, I had the unbelievable luck of hearing, "Caspar Weinberger here."

"Mr. Weinberger, my name is Connie Panzarino. I am a worker for the Department of Social Services in Nassau County, New York. I am disabled and need attendant care to go to the bathroom, make meals, get in and out of bed, bathe and dress. Because your laws say that a person cannot work and still be classified as disabled, I am ineligible for Medicaid benefits to pay for my personal care attendants. Can you help me so that I can go to the bathroom?"

"Miss Panzarino, you are mistaken. Whoever has been giving you information is wrong. Of course you are eligible for attendant care. This government appreciates that people like you are out there working and contributing. Let me have your number and the number of your supervisor and I will take care of this matter immediately."

"Oh, thank you, Mr. Weinberger." I gave him the appropriate numbers and tearfully hung up the phone. "Henry, he said we're wrong, and I *am* eligible."

"I hope he's right." Henry smiled and waggled his finger at me cautionarily. I knew he didn't want me to get hurt from having my hopes dashed.

Later on that afternoon I received a phone call from Mr. Weinberger's secretary. "I'm sorry, but Mr. Weinberger is very busy and asked me to call you to tell you that you are absolutely right, there is no way to provide attendant care for a person who is able to work. He wishes you the best and thanks you for calling."

Next I got a phone call from Mr. Rosa. "Mr. Weinberger's office just called to tell me that we are within our rights in denying you medical assistance. Maybe you can hire a retarded person for ten or twenty dollars a week. You don't need that much help. Anyone could do it."

"Thank you, Mr. Rosa, but no thank you. If a retarded person can be an attendant, they deserve to be paid a full attendant's salary. I'm taking the rest of today off as a personal day."

"I'm sorry," Henry said, his eyes all watery.

Al drove me home on his break. I called my friend Jimmy, Judy Heuman (a woman who had won a suit against the city of New York because they said she could not be a teacher if she was in a wheelchair), Helen from PUSH, Hal Rosenthal from ABCD, and asked them to call every activist they could think of. Judy asked me to come to a meeting with Jimmy to form a coalition of organizations. Disabled In Action of New York grew out of that meeting.

Meanwhile, Mickey was getting tired of waking up every night and groping around for my arms and legs to turn me. I was getting tired of having to see for both of us each morning as she dressed me. All my personal care took at least three times longer. I hired an attendant from an agency with the little money I had in savings. I had only enough for two weeks of personal care. My stomach ulcers reactivated, and I lost weight. When the new attendant found out I only had enough money for two weeks, she quit on the spot. I called Ron's mother and she took me to her house for the night. I woke up with a fever and lung congestion in the morning. I called my doctor to see what I should do.

"Dr. Madonia, I'm pretty sick. I have 102° fever, but I'm afraid to take antibiotics because my ulcers are really acting up. Besides, antibiotics always make me have to go to the bathroom and I don't have an attendant right now."

"What do you mean you don't have an attendant? When's she coming back?"

"Well, you see, I don't have attendant care now because I'm working and I can't share Priscilla's attendant because she doesn't live here anymore so some of my friends have been helping me out, but the law says even if I quit working I'm not eligible because I'm 'able' to work, and I should work, and I don't think I can figure this out right now . . ."

"You are not able to work right now, you have a 102° temperature and I forbid you to go to work. You are under doctor's orders not to work. You send someone back to Medicaid to tell them you are disabled, your doctor says so, and if they want an argument they can see me in court."

The next day Mrs. Kovic took me to the Department of Social Services to hand in my letter of resignation. I applied for and received temporary welfare and Medicaid, and then went to Social Security to apply for permanent disability benefits. Within twenty-four hours I had an attendant, antibiotics, and was back in my own bed.

As soon as my fever went down, I called *Newsday* and told them what had happened. They sent a photographer to document why I needed attendant care. The next day I was on the front page of the paper. There were several pictures of me on the second and third pages showing an attendant transferring me in a Hoyer mechanical lift on and off the bed. My friends and family were furious at the injustice of the law and applauded my fight. Some of my friends with disabilities were appalled that I allowed myself to be shown to the able-bodied public in a vulnerable, dependent position because they felt that it would increase oppression by encouraging the stereotype of the "helpless cripple." I believed that in order to have our needs met we needed to stop trying to "pass" in the able-bodied community and pretend that we were self-reliant because that fed the misconception that attendant care was a frivolity rather than a necessity for life support. The story got picked up by more and more sources and within a week I was on the Channel 4 news.

Legislators, senators, and other government officials began calling me at my home. One U.S. senator offered to write a bill just for me, since I was such an "exception to the rule," allowing me to work and have Medicaid for the rest of my life. I refused because I knew I was no exception. There were many people with disabilities who could work, yet needed attendant care or other medical services which they could not afford on their salaries.

Several weeks later, Disabled In Action sent a contingent of people to a county executive board meeting to confront the Nassau County Executive, Ralph Caso, about not meeting the needs of disabled workers within the county system. This was televised on the three major networks in New York.

I began working with Congressman Mario Biaggi, an ex-policeman with a disability, writing a bill which would allow people with disabilities to work without losing disability status. During that year I assisted in writing eleven local, state and federal bills and policies to attempt to rectify the situation.

Although I eventually received disability benefits of four hundred and fifty dollars per month, it was not enough to pay my rent, food and the upkeep on my car. I was not allowed to accept work or gifts, as this would jeopardize my Medicaid status.

Chris, one of Ron's old girlfriends, had been following my story. She offered to move in with me as a roommate, share the rent, and work as my attendant. She took the ten weeks of training required by Medicaid, registered with the appropriate agency, and wore a white uniform, required by law, while she took care of me. Chris was a financial and emotional support.

The phone began to ring constantly. There were four or five people writing letters or reading bills or meeting with me every afternoon. Our home quickly took on the atmosphere of a central office for a grassroots movement for workers with disabilities.

14

TRENDELENBURG

Ron moved to California for several months. He could afford it since he received one hundred and fifty percent disability from the VA plus a large Social Security check each month. It was quite a sum of money to live on. Sometimes he enjoyed it, sometimes he flaunted it, but most of the time he wasted it in disgust calling it "blood money." He was always coming and going. It mostly felt like going, but the comings were so wonderful that I always waited for him like a faithful sailor's wife.

Ron began writing a book about his life telling what the Vietnam War was like for him. I was thrilled because he was finally writing the book I had dreamed he would write. I felt it was important that the truth about the insanity of the war be told and that young people never again be duped into going to war. I gave Ron all the support I could, even listening when he called me collect from a pay phone to read me the entire six hundred-page manuscript. My phone bill was seven hundred and fifty dollars that month. Ron paid some of the bill and I set up a payment plan with the phone company to pay off the rest.

"Hey Babe! Roger and I are at the Chelsea Hotel in New York. He says we're going to sell my book. How are you? I'm freezing. I got my California T-shirt and jeans on and it can't be more than twenty-five degrees out. Can you help us out?"

"Sure. It's 11 P.M. now, give me an hour or so to pack up and another hour to drive in. I'll be there around one, okay?"

"Great, Connie. You're great. I love you."

"I love you too. See you soon." I hung up the phone and turned to Chris. "Hurray! The book's done. He's in town with Roger. They're at the Chelsea. He says there's hardly any heat, and tons of roaches, but I guess the atmosphere makes up for it. Let's pack a bunch of warm stuff for them and go join the party." Chris and I packed up our clothes as well as warm sweaters, long underwear and wool socks for Ron and Roger. We took the hot pot, instant coffee, tea, hot chocolate and tunafish sandwiches. On the way in we stopped at a 24-hour store and bought a small heater. We spent several days at the hotel.

Ron read me a new chapter he had written, telling how in the confusion of a Vietcong ambush and the chaos of young men screaming in anguish, he mistakenly killed an American soldier in his platoon. He sobbed into my arms afterward. "Do you still love me? How can you love me when I've done such a terrible thing?"

I held him close. "It's okay, Ron. I've known about the ambush from your flashbacks. I've known for a long time and loved you anyway." We held each other and made love that night.

The next day, Ron sold his book, *Born on the Fourth of July*, to McGraw-Hill. We celebrated with a big dinner, champagne and lovemaking. In the middle of the night he woke up burning up with fever. I took him home to my apartment on Long Island. The next morning it turned out he had the flu, and within several days, Chris, her boyfriend Louis and I had 104° temperatures. The agency sent attendant after attendant to care for me because Chris was too sick to work. They all came down with the flu, which was rapidly spreading throughout New York. Some of them left because it was too much work.

One aide walked out on me at four in the morning and left me upside down over a pillow coughing. Ron helped me turn on my back, and shouted for Chris, who was nearly unconscious in the other room. Then Ron sponge-bathed me with alcohol to bring down my fever and we both fell asleep naked. The next morning at eight my mother came in to see if we needed help. She was horrified at the two of us lying there naked in each other's arms. My brother later told me that when she came home, she threw up and screamed and cried. I don't know why—maybe because we weren't married, or because we both had twisted, disabled bodies, or because she felt helpless and sorry for us. She didn't have to worry that I'd become pregnant, because Ron was infertile. I was too sick at the time to talk about my mother's reaction, but it hurt me for a long time.

Ron and I had been living in the same bed for nearly two weeks, becoming like prisoners sharing a jail cell. Ron's mother came in one day, grabbed all the sheets, towels and blankets, and took them to the laundromat. She left us with one blanket. Ron began to write poetry on the mattress and we played tic-tac-toe until the laundry came back. We nearly froze before she returned. Kathy came and tried to cook us some food, but I was too sick to eat.

The man from the surgical supply place came and brought me a respirator to ease my breathing and clear the congestion in my lungs. Ron called him the "Respirator Man." The sound of the respirator freaked Ron out because he had heard it so often in the hospital. I grew worse and worse, as did Ron, Louis and Chris. I went to the hospital emergency room three times because I could barely breathe. They suctioned my lungs to clear them out, but they wouldn't keep me because there weren't enough beds. Over the last several weeks the flu had become an epidemic of such magnitude that they closed the universities. That night, my cousin Carol, who had never taken care of me before, came to help me because the agency was short-handed due to the epidemic. She was wonderful.

The next morning, the Public Health nurse came and arranged for Chris and Louis to go to their parents' houses to recuperate. She sent Ron to the VA hospital because he was developing a kidney infection as a result of the flu. She called an ambulance for me and arranged for a room at the hospital.

It was snowing hard when the ambulance came. They refused to put a blanket over me when we went out into the street because they were afraid they would trip on the blanket in the snow. I got covered with snow as they carried me around the corner to where the ambulance was parked. Carol kept yelling at them to cover me with a blanket, but they wouldn't. I was too weak to talk above a whisper. After I got into the ambulance, they finally put a blanket over me, causing all the snow on me to melt and making me wet and cold. Oddly enough they didn't know the way to the hospital, and my cousin was from New Jersey so she couldn't help them. I was too sick to figure out where we were, especially since I couldn't see much out the windows. We drove around Long Island for an hour. When we reached the hospital, I waited four or five hours for a bed, shivering on a stretcher in an alcove in the hall. My mother came and sat in a chair by my feet. Carol sat on another stretcher.

They put me in a regular ward with a private duty nurse who was paid fifty dollars per shift. That afternoon, Medicaid determined that they would not pay for the private duty nurse. The hospital said my parents also refused because they could not afford it. The doctors had no choice but to put me in the intensive care unit (ICU) because the nursing staff said they could not handle my level of physical need. I wanted to tell my parents that I hated them. I wanted to die to spite them all—Medicaid, my parents, the ambulance drivers, and the nurses who didn't know how to take care of me. But I decided to live to spite them.

Everyone around me was unconscious and on loud, beeping machines. I was fighting for each breath. I could not even lay down to sleep because I would choke. But I desperately needed to sleep since I had not slept in days.

The nurses were never supposed to leave the ICU untended. At least one nurse was supposed to be in the room at all times, but that didn't happen. They would take their coffee breaks together and hang out in the halls, laughing and telling stories. They resented me because I was conscious and knew they were breaking the rules, and because I wasn't as sick as the others in the room. When I needed them to reposition me because I couldn't breathe, they tried to suction me instead. The suctioning didn't work since my trachea was not straight like most people's. They could have used smaller, more flexible child-sized suctioning tubes, but instead they used adult-sized tubes which tore up my throat and caused me to bleed and gag more. It felt like behavior modification gone wild. If I didn't complain I could choke and die, but if I did complain and they suctioned me, I could choke and die from the suctioning. I learned to hate in the ICU as I had never hated in my life.

I was only allowed visitors for fifteen minutes three times a day. Ron only came once. He thought I was going to die, so he freaked out and took off for California. Mom or Dad came once a day. I could barely look them in the eye, I was so angry with them for not paying for a private duty nurse. I thought it was their fault I was there. They had a boat and a Cadillac. How could they say they couldn't afford a couple of hundred dollars a day? I was too weak to argue it out with them. I was too weak to tell them they should fight with Medicaid.

Maybe my mom and dad and Ron gave up on me and didn't want to invest in me. Maybe they were scared. It was the first time I ever realized how similar Ron was to my mother. They both treated me like I was the most precious thing on earth at times, and then at other times wanted to run the other way. I never knew whether Ron was mean to me because of what the war did to him, because of his up-bringing or because he resented my disability. When my mother was mean to me, I never knew whether it was be-cause of who she was and her problems, or my disability. But I was physically more depleted than I had ever been in my life, and emotionally more drained as well. I knew I could never think of depending upon my parents for survival ever again. I had realized that before, for brief moments, but now I was sure. I knew I couldn't trust Ron either. I felt very alone.

One nurse accidently gave me peroxide to drink instead of water. Twice they put Tylenol suppositories in my vagina instead of my anus. They ignored me when I told them it was the wrong opening, then checked grudgingly. I would cry out endlessly to be moved and turned because the pres-sure of being in one position caused such pain. They would yell at me to shut up and tell me they had to take care of sick people. My vision blurred and my hearing got muffled. My taste buds were so deadened that I put six lumps of sugar in the decaffeinated coffee they gave me one day, and couldn't taste it. I thought I was dying. No one told me that many of my symptoms were side effects of the strong antibiotics and decongestants I was being given.

Through it all, I kept fighting. I contracted two secondary respiratory infections on top of the flu. When I was finally getting better, a nurse who was taking care of me began coughing in my face. I asked her if she was sick. She said she had a 102° temperature. I told her to get away from me and not to touch me because I didn't want to get sick and die. She told me that she had children at home and had to work because she needed the money. I wept in frustration. Forty-eight hours later I had 104° temperature and pneumonia.

I spent most of the next few days on my stomach in "Trendelenburg"—a position with the bed tilted so that my head was lower than my feet. That way gravity could help the lung secretions drain out of me. I felt very alone, but I did not feel ready to give up. I told God that I was going to live in spite of him.

They brought a new woman in and put her next to me. She had overdosed and had been in a coma for several months. Her family came in three times a day and tried to talk her out of her coma. Then they brought in tapes of her little girl crying for her mommy. "Mommy! Mommy! Please wake up. I need you Mommy. Please wake up!" The nurses kept putting it on over and over, and once they left the tape on all night. The next night they left a radio on. I thought I would go mad.

They put me in a room by myself with a TV for one blessed evening. It was wonderful, except I was afraid to be so alone since my fingers weren't strong enough to push the button to call for the nurse. My lungs were beginning to clear. I had been working hard on coughing, drinking fluids and visualizing clear air space in my lungs. I was beginning to sleep for nearly an hour at a time. Chris, as soon as she was able, came to visit me twice a day. When I was too afraid to sleep, she lay next to me and held me so I could sleep for the fifteen minute visiting period. It felt safe to sleep that way because if I stopped breathing she would wake me up. I gained strength.

I was transferred to another ICU, for less traumatically injured people. In the new unit the nurses were wonderful. The few times that I had to wait for a bedpan, or to get turned in bed, they apologized and explained who they had taken care of and what had happened. They often took time to offer me tea or juice. In the other unit I'd had to beg for water. The last night I was in the new unit, they called and ordered pizza for me. They seemed to like me, and they liked their work.

I was discharged from the hospital, but I still wasn't well. I had to use a respirator twice a day. Breathing in and out on it exhausted me. My life changed from being an activist to watching soap operas and old TV movies in my pajamas. It felt weird, but I had to do it because I was still recovering. A lot of my disabled friends didn't have jobs because if they worked they'd lose their disability benefits. I saw them becoming depressed as their lives centered around playing solitaire or watching TV, and was afraid that this would happen to me.

I kept fighting for the right to work because I knew I would get well eventually, and I wanted to be allowed to work then. On September 11, 1974, I sent a mailgram to President Ford:

> Incapable of toileting, bathing, dressing myself—penalized for working full time. Income from employment insufficient for home health aide's salary. Ineligible for medicaid—person working full-time earning over $140 per month not considered federally disabled. Forced to resign 8/22/74 to qualify for Welfare/SSI/Medicaid and have home health aid. Sentenced to life of dependency. Request for presidential pardon to permit my return to work while maintaining home health aid under partial medicaid as disabled person. Signed Miss Connie Panzarino

I figured that as long as he had pardoned Nixon, he could pardon me, but I never heard from him. I began a lawsuit through Legal Aid Services against Nassau County, New York State, and Caspar Weinberger, the Secretary of Health, Education and Welfare. The lawsuit held him responsible for my job loss. I hoped the court would rule that the definition of disability, which was solely based on one's ability to earn money, would be declared unconstitutional, and that I would then be reinstated at my job, but with full attendant care benefits.

I didn't see too much of my sister except at family gatherings. My brother and I became close. I think he liked to come and stay over at his big sister's apartment. My sister couldn't really do that without my mother there to meet her personal needs. I also think that my hospitalization terrified Pidgie. When I saw her at big Sunday family dinners she would chitchat about school, but she didn't really ask me much about what I was doing. It felt like she was afraid to know how I was feeling or what was happening.

Ron came back sheepishly, and asked me to marry him. I didn't really take him seriously because his moods and life-style were so changeable, but said yes, just in case he really meant it. We had a turkey dinner to celebrate and Ron carved the turkey. He asked Louis to be his permanent aide. He said that way the four of us could all live together. Two days later Ron decided he liked life as a bachelor, and left for California, taking Louis with him.

I found out through Judy Heuman that disabled people in California were sometimes able to work and keep some of their attendant care. Since I had been so ill that winter I liked the idea of living where it was warmer. I no longer felt the need to live close to my family since the hospital experience had showed me that they would not always be there for me when I needed them.

Chris was missing Louis, and I was missing Ron, so we decided to move to California. When we figured out our travel expenses, we were short two hundred and fifty dollars each. Chris and I decided to sell our bodies to medical science to raise the money. We called the local hospital at 2 A.M. to ask how we could do this. The woman who answered was quite amazed and asked why it was such an emergency and couldn't we please wait until the next morning? When we called the next morning, we found out that they paid two hundred and fifty dollars per body, but that most bodies that are bought lie around in big vats in medical schools for years and years with hundreds of other dead bodies. We didn't feel comfortable with that so we decided against it. Luckily we found a special on airfare to California, so we were no longer short the money. We sold all our furniture and packed up my car with everything I owned including the wooden ramps from my apartment. Pete, a friend of ours who had cerebral palsy, agreed to drive it all out there. A week after he left, Chris and I flew to Los Angeles.

When we landed, Shannon, the friend of Ron's I had met on my first trip to California, and her baby, Zephyr, were waiting for us. Pete was there with my car, right on schedule. Louis had found an apartment, but it was up two flights of steps so we couldn't take it. Louis was at work and would meet us at his apartment that afternoon.

"I put all your stuff in Louis' apartment for the time being so there would be room for you in the car, okay? He said you can keep it there if you want to until you find a place of your own." Pete smiled his twisted smile and ruffled up my hair.

"Well, Bob and I are staying with Ron's friend Jeannie and her two kids in Santa Monica. Jeannie's from New York. I'm sure there's plenty of room there, it's a two-bedroom apartment. Plus there's a big king-sized bed in the living room and lots of pillows on the floor. Why don't you stay there with us?" Shannon smiled.

"Great," I said. We all piled into the car and off we went.

On the way to Jeannie's we stopped off at Louis' and left him a note with Jeannie's address and asked him to meet us there after work. When we got to Jeannie's, she met us with a big New York hug and lots of reminiscent talk. When we went inside, I was impressed with the size of the waterbed, but the apartment was small.

Somehow we managed. Ron and Louis joined us there. Eight adults and three children stayed in that apartment for the two weeks it took for us to get jobs and find places to live. One night we had six people sleeping on the waterbed. The phone rang constantly, and each mealtime was like a party.

I found an apartment and installed the ramps that I had taken from my old apartment in New York. The Bible students in California helped me get furniture. Chris helped me put my apartment together and interview attendants. I hired a woman named Julie. She was from Australia. Chris agreed to work with Julie for two weeks to train her in my routine care.

One night Ron was out of town, Chris and Louis were staying over, and Julie, the new attendant, was working. I suggested that Chris and Louis take my double bed, Julie sleep in the living room, and I sleep in the attendant's room on the single bed. Everyone agreed and we all went to sleep. In the middle of the night I called out, "Julie? Julie! I need to be turned."

In the shadows I saw her turning the knob to go into the room where Chris and Louis were sleeping. "Julie!" I whispered. "I'm in here."

"Be quiet, Connie. I have to turn Chris over." I watched Julie turn the doorknob and go into my bedroom, where Chris was sleeping with Louis.

As she turned back the covers to turn Chris, Chris sat bolt upright in bed. "Oh, I'm sorry, Julie. Did I call you?"

Julie immediately became embarrassed. "No, no. Never mind." Julie went back to bed.

I began laughing. Sometimes attendants do the strangest things in the middle of the night. I remembered several times when Chris had slept so soundly that our neighbor upstairs would hear me calling for her, and would dial our number so the ringing phone would wake Chris up.

Chris and Louis were fighting a lot. She felt he had changed since he had been in California. He was not working for Ron anymore. He got a job driving a bus and seemed happy, but Chris was homesick. She found herself unwilling to commit to a long-term relationship with Louis, so she decided to go back to New York as soon as I was settled.

The California attendant care system was different than

in New York. The attendant care check went directly to me, and it was my responsibility to find and pay attendants. This was better, because I could hire and train whomever I chose, but the maximum amount allowable was five hundred dollars per month, which was less than twenty dollars per day. In New York, my attendants had been getting thirty-five per day.

I hired several aides, but they only stayed short periods of time. Some stayed a day, some stayed a month. Sometimes they left because the pay was so low. Other times they left because they were in transition themselves. Some said they left because they were uncomfortable with how erratic my days and nights were because of my living with Ron. As he rewrote his book, his mood swings and flashbacks increased.

"No! No! Stop! Stop!" Ron ducked down in his chair and covered his head.

I went over to him and talked softly. "Ronnie, it's okay. You're home now. It's over. You're not there anymore. The war's over." I waited, not daring to touch him for fear of triggering a violent response.

Ron's breathing changed, his arms dropped down limply and he looked at me, stunned. He started weeping and leaned over to put his head in my lap. "When will it stop, Babe? When will it stop!"

"I don't know, Ronnie, but I know it will stop some day. Why don't you get some sleep? You've been up all night writing, haven't you?"

"Yeah." Ron sat up in his chair and looked at me. "Could you hear me pounding the keys? I keep trying to write about boot camp, but it's tough, you know? It's real tough."

"I know, Ronnie, I know. But it's going to be a great book. Let me read that chapter again."

"I took out a lot of the details, it was getting too long."

"No, Ron. You've got to stop worrying about the length. I know it's painful for you to put it all down on paper, but Joyce will edit whatever is extra. I think you need to put more in about the sergeant. Are you hungry?"

"Nah. I think I need to get some sleep. I'll see you in a few hours. Maybe we can go to the beach. Would you like that? Would you like to go to the beach with me?"

"Yeah, that'd be great. You get some sleep, I'm going to have some breakfast." I hugged and kissed him and he went off to the bedroom.

I looked around me at the living room. There were three dirty coffee cups, one laying on its side with a pool of coffee around it. There were piles of crumpled paper on the floor from failed attempts at writing the chapter. Cigarette butts were everywhere, a banana peel was cascading down the back of the couch, a half-eaten apple was on the window sill, and a piece of unwrapped cheese was sitting next to the typewriter. I turned to Terry, my attendant, and said, "Let's clean up before we have breakfast."

Terry was a male nurse who had taken the Monday through Friday daytime position. At night and on weekends I had a student named Martha who took care of me in exchange for free room and board, plus twenty-five dollars per day in spending money. This arrangement had worked for a little over a month so far.

After breakfast, I went to the store and came back, hoping Ron would wake up so we could go to the beach. I read the pages he had written the night before and wept at their intensity. I made some editorial notations and corrected some of the grammar and spelling. I ate some fruit and played with my cat and hoped Ron would wake up. I didn't want to wake him because I knew how exhausted he was. I didn't want to go to the beach without him, but I was bored and missing him.

At five that evening I made dinner with Terry. He left at six and Martha took over. Ron woke up and came to give me a big hug. We discussed the writing he had done the night before and then he went to take a bath.

"I made spaghetti for dinner," I shouted after him.

"Great! I'm starved. I'll be there in a few minutes."

Half an hour later Ron came whizzing through the living room smelling of soap and shaving lotion. "How do I look?"

"Great! Ready for dinner?"

"I'm not hungry. I'm going to go shoot pool for a while. I'll see you later." He zipped out the door.

I sighed and sat at the table to eat dinner with Martha. I ached for him in his pain and tried to comfort myself in my own. None of the Vietnam vets that I knew were having an easy time in their relationships. Last week Bob had hit Shannon right in front of Zephyr, and then freaked out and wanted to kill himself for what he had done. The guys that hadn't died over there had come home to live in their own private hell.

After dinner I went to the beach and walked on the boardwalk. I came home around nine and found Ron throwing up in the bathroom. He was sobbing about killing babies and old people in a hut. The typewriter was out and there was crumpled up paper strewn everywhere.

"It's okay, Ronnie, it's okay." I went into the bathroom and had Martha lift my arm around Ron's shoulder. "You're fine, Ronnie, I'm here."

Martha and I helped Ron get into the tub to wash off. When he got out of the tub, he ate some dinner and told me about another chapter he was working on. I went over his writing and made comments and suggestions in the margin. At 11:30 P.M. I said, "I'm beat, Ron. I have to get some sleep."

"Sure, Babe. I'm going to write for a little bit and I'll be in soon." He kissed me good night and I went to bed.

At three in the morning Ron fell into bed, exhausted, with all his clothes on, and went to sleep. He tossed and turned in the fit of a nightmare. About an hour later I woke up, drenched with warm wet liquid. I was exhausted. The room smelled of urine. I hated it. Ron had been too tired to hook up his overnight urinary drainage bag. During his nightmare, the overly full leg-bag had pulled loose, its contents emptying completely onto the bed. I felt bad for Ron. I hated to wake him up. I knew he'd be more upset than I was, and it pained me to hear him complain. I was sorry for him, sorry for me, and most of all sorry for my attendant.

"Martha! The bed is wet."

Martha came sleepily into the room. "This is the third time this week." She lifted me out of the bed and carried me to the living room couch. Ron woke up in the process and began cursing and swearing about the war and leg-bags and piss and shit. He hooked up his overnight leg-bag and settled himself on pillows on the living room floor.

The next morning, Terry put the mattress out in the sun and washed all the sheets and bedclothes with bleach. It was a lot of work for an aide to keep up with Ron's extremes and my needs. Sometimes I was afraid they would leave. Sometimes they did leave, and I had to go through the stress of hiring and training all over again.

The rest of the week was no better. Ron eventually finished the chapter about his platoon shooting a hut full of children. He sobbed in my arms for over an hour after he finished the chapter.

All of a sudden he sat upright in his chair and pushed me away. "How can you love someone like me? What are you, sick? You must be sick! I'm a murderer, don't you understand? A murderer. How can you be with a murderer? God, what am I going to do? I'm a murderer!"

"Ronnie, stop it!" I couldn't get through to him. He wouldn't let me touch him and he wouldn't listen to me or look me in the eye. He went down the hall and I heard the bedroom door slam. I started to cry. Terry came into the room to be available if I needed him.

A short time later, Ron came back into the room with Martha. He told me that he and Martha were going to New York together because they were in love. I was furious and devastated. I fell apart for the next few days and got a lot of comfort from many of Ron's friends. Terry stayed with me day and night.

A week later, Martha came back and apologized. She said she hated Ron and would never understand how I'd been with him so long and how I'd put up with him. She said she never wanted to see him again and was glad to be home. I fired her on the spot and told her to leave my house.

Ron and I walked a tightrope between passion and hatred. He was raw from the war, and I was trying to be the good wife he never really wanted. When I wasn't being "the good wife," and I was being myself, he loved me much more. When he could get beyond his guilt of having been used in the war machine to kill and maim, we laughed and played and planned together. Once I dyed my hair blond, thinking it would please him. He laughed and said he loved my brown hair and hated that I kept trying to change myself. He didn't like women to wear makeup. I didn't understand him. I thought men liked women who wore makeup.

California was the first place where men came on to me sexually. It didn't seem to matter that I was in a wheelchair. I found this delightful, but I always refused them. My rationale was that since I was a Christian I shouldn't have intercourse unless I was married. Even though I was living with Ron, we weren't having intercourse, so that seemed all right.

Ron, though, often had sexual relationships with other women. At first I felt hurt. I thought I wasn't good enough to satisfy him because I was disabled—it seemed like he had to have sex with able-bodied women who could wrestle with him in bed. When I wasn't being jealous, I felt loved and valued because his relationships with the able-bodied women never lasted more than a year or two at most and usually only lasted a few weeks, while his relationship with me was constant.

Ron encouraged me to go out with other men since he had other girlfriends. I wasn't really interested. He also encouraged me to have relationships with women. Our friend Shannon was bisexual and often had female lovers in addition to her relationship with Bob. I thought he was crazy. I refused to even think about being involved with anyone else but Ron.

While I was in California, I spent a lot of time looking for employment. Since all my experience doing Social Service referrals had been in New York, none of the agencies were willing to take the time to train and orient me to the California Social Services system. I went to the California State Vocational Rehabilitation Commission to be re-evaluated for employment training.

During the three months it took for the Vocational Rehabilitation re-evaluation, I began to sell some of the artwork that I had done over the years. I began to paint and draw more and more. What had been a recreational tool for me was becoming profitable. I had often given my art work as gifts to relatives and friends, but had never taken myself seriously as an artist before.

I tried not to be discouraged about not working. Terry had become more than an attendant. He was an invaluable friend. He could tell when I was getting down and feeling like a useless cripple, or when I felt overwhelmed at all the barriers that appeared to surround me or when I began creating chaos in my life to distract me from my fears. At those moments he would whisk me off to see a sunset or a movie, or grab a fishing pole shouting, "Quick, Connie! There's a big fish waiting at the end of the Santa Monica pier for us. I can see him. If we hurry, we can have him for dinner." Terry would have me out the door and in the car in spite of my half-hearted protests. Over time I learned to be good to myself and have fun, especially when things were hard. I bought a button to wear that said, "Living well is the best revenge."

Occasionally I sat outside in the driveway of the apartment building where Ron and I lived. Kids who lived in the
building would watch me draw, and sometimes I would draw
pictures of them. I began to organize art projects that we
would do together. Sometimes I walked them all to the park
or the store. I think they liked me because I was different. I
liked them because they were open, energetic and accepting
of me.

One little girl in particular, Dawn, became very special to
me. Her parents were divorced, although still living together for financial reasons. Both her parents suffered from
mental illness at the time and had little energy left for
Dawn. She was six years old and very quick. She was the
only child I ever met who accepted me and my disability totally. She sat on my lap and we told each other stories.
Dawn often ate in my home and slept there if her parents
were out. When she was outside playing she often came in
to see if I had been calling her, or if I was lonely. We had
fun together. We would paint each other's fingernails and
put flowers in our hair. Sometimes we would go to the park
and have ice cream picnics.

I had always wanted to have children. I had been told that
I could bear children, but would probably have to spend the
last few months of pregnancy in bed. I knew that Ron and I
could never have children, but we talked about adopting, or
artificial insemination. My biggest fear about having children, though, was not directly because of my disability, but
because I would have to rely on attendants to take care of a
child, and it was difficult to trust attendants in such a sensitive area. Once I'd had a kitten who was allergic to milk. I
told all my attendants to never give her milk. Three times in
six months, attendants snuck her milk in spite of what I had
directed. Each time the kitten almost died. "What would
have happened if that had been my child?" I thought to myself.

Dawn filled my need for having a child of my own. I believed that the odds of my having one that would be as close to me as she already was were very small. After all, many of the children around me seemed so disinterested in their natural parents, and many parents seemed estranged from their children. I decided not to have a child of my own and to put my financial and emotional energy into Dawn's upbringing while always being careful to support her relationship with her real parents, because they did love her and they were her natural parents.

Grandma came to visit for her seventy-fifth birthday. She told all the relatives that she was coming to California to take me home. She just told me she was coming to visit for a week.

She loved the sun and the water. She said it reminded her of Sicily. She was getting on in years and was having more and more trouble with the circulation in her legs. At night they would burn and she could not sleep from the pain.

One night at eleven o'clock, just as the news was finishing, I said, "Okay, Gram, get your sweater. We're going to go for a walk."

"Whadda you, craze? Itsa tima go ta sleepa."

"No! You're not going to sleep anyway. Let's go look at the water. Terry, get the car."

"I'm already on my way out the door, Connie." Terry jangled the car keys up in the air and went out.

We drove to the Marina del Ray pier and walked out over the water under the stars for nearly an hour. The sound of the waves was hypnotic. Pretty soon we were all yawning. We went home and went to bed.

The next morning Grandma woke up before me and started cooking in the kitchen. Terry got me up. I went into the kitchen to find Grandma humming and dancing around. "How'd you sleep, Gram?"

"I sleepa fine. My legsa no bahda me. I lika California."

Grandma stayed three weeks, which was the longest she could stay with her airline ticket. Every night we went for a long walk on the pier, and every day we went sightseeing. She cooked up a storm of Italian delights for me and Terry and half the neighborhood.

"Grandma, what are you making?" shouted Patty, my upstairs neighbor as she came home from work.

"Cappanadine!" Grandma looked at Patty with a grin. "Eggaplanta with olives and a sausa. You wanna some?"

Patty came in and sat down. Billy from next door came in with a bag of groceries. "Here, Grandma, I bought tomatoes and mozzarella so you can make pizza for us tomorrow."

Grandma seemed to make friends with everyone in the building.

I took her to Disneyland. We got there when it opened and left at one in the morning when the park closed. We went to Universal Studios. We went on the tram that takes you through an avalanche. Grandma screamed and began to make the sign of the cross, "Gesú Christo! Connie! Why you taka me ona these things? I'ma olla lady." When the day was over, Grandma wanted to come back and do the ride again! Grandma and I had a good time, and I hated to see her leave. It was hard not to get on the plane with her.

I hadn't found a job so I went to the California State Vocational Rehabilitation Office to discuss the results of their evaluation. They suggested that I get my Masters in art therapy. I had never heard of art therapy before, so I began reading about it and exploring programs across the country that offered it. It appeared to be a field that would suit me. I began to get excited about going back to school.

In the meantime, I was having more and more difficulty keeping attendants, and had become homesick for my friends and family in New York.

Chris came out to visit me for a few days, courtesy of

Ron. I decided to leave California and go back with her to New York. There were better art therapy programs in New York, and the attendant care system was a little better there. I also wanted to pursue my court case to regain the right to work, and I could not do that from California.

Dawn was heartbroken. I explained to her as best I could why I was leaving, and gave her as many of my things as I could so that she would have tangible evidence that I cared for her. A friend of ours, Tony, agreed to stay and pack up all my belongings and drive my car to New York. He told me that Dawn came in to visit him several days after I left, while he was still packing my things. She was looking very sad. She asked him if he missed me, and if he was sad. He said "Yes." She asked him what he liked to do when he was sad. He said he didn't know, then asked her what she liked to do when she was sad. She said she liked to dance and would he please dance with her. They danced in my empty apartment in my honor. Dawn left laughing.

15

WHO'S WEARING
THE PANTS?

I took some graduate courses at Hofstra University that combined the fields of psychology and art, and read several books by Edith Kramer. The more I learned about art therapy, the more I liked it. I enjoyed working with and helping people, and I enjoyed making art. Art therapy seemed a more powerful and painless way to provide psychotherapy than conventional talk-therapy. Using images as metaphors was almost like working directly with the unconscious, and it was fun for both the client and the therapist.

Ron and I were living in an apartment in Hempstead. His book had been published, and he was beginning to try to get it made into a movie. His moods were more erratic than ever, and he was often away for months at a time. Sometimes he would go out to do a fifteen minute errand and come back two weeks later, having flown to Paris, Ireland, or Los Angeles in the meantime. I became increasingly angry and felt more and more depressed each time he left.

One of my attendants, Maura, became a primary support to me at this time. Maura was a lesbian. I had been afraid of hiring lesbians because I had been told by my mother and other disabled friends that lesbians attacked women with disabilities. Nothing could have been further from the truth. It was Maura who helped me to feel confident in myself and safe with others.

"How's your paper going, Connie?"

"I don't know if I'll ever get it done, Maura."

"Sure you will! Just be patient, it's a big project. Did you make an appointment with that lawyer you heard about?"

"Yeah, Curtis Brewer. I have an appointment next week, but I'm pretty scared about going. My case has been rejected by so many lawyers, I don't know if I can keep trying. I think I should just forget it."

"It's been really hard for you, and I don't blame you if you need to stop, but this lawyer might be really different because he's disabled. You have a right to work and a right to fight for your rights. I'm sorry it's been so hard. Have you heard from Ron today?"

"No."

"Well, I'm sure you'll hear from him. It's really not fair, the way he's treating you right now, but I'm sure it'll get better."

Maura was the only person I had met up to that point who maintained a positive attitude and who believed in me even when I felt unsure of myself. Through her I learned that disabled women are oppressed in this culture not only because they are disabled, but also because they are women. A far higher percentage of disabled men were given education through the state Rehabilitation Commission than were women.

One night Maura was helping her sister move furniture when she hurt her back. She could no longer be my attendant and could not work for several years after that. She couldn't pay rent, and didn't want to move back to her mother's house, so I asked her if she wanted to stay with me for a while. After all, Ron was gone so much of the time, I was a bit lonely for company and Maura and I were both artists. I thought it would be nice to have someone with whom I could paint and draw. Maura moved in the next day and set up a daybed at one end of the living room.

Maura pursued her healing by seeing doctors and doing back exercises and meditation, while I pursued my studies in art and psychology. I took a five week intensive course on sexuality, which required that I keep a journal about feelings that came up in relation to what we were learning in class. I began to realize that what was coming up for me in class about sexuality had to do with women. I became anxious because I was nauseated by the films showing intercourse. I could not imagine fondling or having oral sex with a penis. On the other hand, I saw vulvas as beautiful. I shared my perceptions with Maura who validated me completely. She began to do four-by-five foot paintings of vulva flower-like abstracts.

I filled my journal with pages and pages of description of how beautiful Lois, my former babysitter, had been, and how I still had dreams of Mrs. Sullivan holding me and kissing me. I wrote about my friend Susie, who had never married, and had been living with a woman for many years. I wrote about all the gay men I found myself attracted to. I wrote about my cousin Gloria who had also never married and was rumored to be lesbian, although no one ever asked her and she never said anything about it. I wrote about how Gloria and I sat together at family weddings, and how I fantasized about dancing with her.

Ron came home after being away for two months. "Hi, Babe, it's good to be home. I'm going to take a bath and change. Can I borrow a pair of your pants?"

"The last three pairs of pants you borrowed, I haven't seen since. I don't want to lend you any more until you replace them. Do you want to go shopping for some clothes today?"

"Look, uh, why don't I just give you twenty dollars and you can give me a pair of your pants." Ron smiled and gave me an affectionate squeeze.

"How about paying me for your share of the last two months' rent first?" I blew him a kiss.

"Oh yeah, here." He tossed a wad of money on the bed

and grabbed a pair of my pants out of the drawer.

"Ron! Just because you have money doesn't mean you can have my clothes whenever you want them."

Ron finished putting my pants on himself and headed out the door. "See you later, Babe."

When he came back that night, I was angry. "Where've you been? I thought maybe we would have dinner together."

"Would you get over it and stop being so old-fashioned? We're not married, and even if we were, I'm not the type to be home for dinner every night, and you shouldn't be the type of woman that stays home and cooks. Haven't you ever heard of women's liberation?"

"Haven't you ever heard of men's liberation, like being independent enough to have your own clothes? Why can't you take some responsibility for communicating with me?"

Maura walked past our room to go to the bathroom. Ron glanced at her with disdain. "What's she still doing here anyway? You told me a month ago she was going to stay with you for a while. Why is she still staying here if I'm paying half the rent? What's she doing here anyway?"

"I don't know," I said quietly. I thought about my journal and the women, and how I loved the way Maura tossed her hair back with her hand. I loved her blue eyes, her smile and her caring.

"Well, I want her to leave, right now."

"Forget it, she's not going anywhere. You're never here anyway. I'm tired of being your doormat. I'm tired of feeling like I'm not good enough and I'm tired of being used. When you're sick or you're freaked out or you happen to be in New York, then you come home to me. I want consistency in our relationship."

"Fine. Then you can both leave. This is my apartment, I'm on the lease."

"Like hell! I'm on the lease too, so we'll divide the apartment in half. I'll sleep in the living room and you can have the bedroom. I'll see you later, I have to go to class now."

When I got back from class, all of Ron's belongings were gone, including two more pairs of my pants. I started to cry. Maura came in, saying, "I'm sorry, Connie. Maybe he'll come back. I know you really love him." She put her arms around me and held me.

"I'm not crying because I'm going to miss him. I'm crying because I feel good that he's gone, and I can't believe I kept looking for love for so long from someone who was so incapable of giving it to me. I began to feel sorry for him, and that's no basis for a relationship."

Tears welled up in my eyes and spilled over. I felt grief for myself growing up as a girl, thinking that my very being depended upon whether I could become a wife. I thought that if I could become a wife, it meant I could be a mother, and being a mother meant I could have power like my mother. I sobbed because I felt like damaged goods. My mind was flooded with images of my mother wanting more of me, wanting more from me, and rejecting me, like Ron and Glenn and Jimmy. It all felt the same.

Suddenly something clicked for me. I realized that other women felt like this too, even if they weren't disabled. I remembered comforting many beautiful able-bodied women who were having struggles with their boyfriends or fights with their mothers. As I sobbed I began to feel strong and angry. I didn't want to worship someone. I wanted an equal relationship. I began to feel sorry for my mother. I think she did a lot more work than my father, and yet he seemed to need all the attention. She probably wasn't able to teach me how to have an equal relationship because she didn't think I could even have a relationship. Or maybe it was because growing up in the thirties and forties, she had never learned to have an equal relationship herself. I just knew that I wanted one, or I didn't want one at all, not with her, or a man or anyone.

Maura just held me.

· · ·

Maura got disability benefits and helped me pay the rent. She began dating a woman in Brooklyn. She talked about going back to school and possibly needing to move to Brooklyn. I began having erotic dreams about her.

At that time my weekend aide was a young college art student named Susan. One Friday when she came in for her shift she burst into tears and asked to talk to Maura. Maura came in and sat with us as Susan sobbed, "I'm in love with my best friend, who is a woman. I don't know what to do about it. I'm scared."

I listened with open ears. Maura said warmly, "That's wonderful that you know you have those feelings. You don't have to be afraid of them because you don't have to do anything about them except feel them. You don't have to be a lesbian, it doesn't mean you are. You don't have to tell the woman or change your life in any way, unless you want to. If you want to, you can. Maybe the woman will be open and maybe she won't, but you aren't a bad person for having those feelings. We all love women in some ways and they aren't any more wrong or right than other ways."

They talked for about an hour and I was very quiet. Afterwards I took Susan down to the mailroom and burst into hysterical tears. "I've been so jealous about Maura and so terrified about what I'll do when she leaves because I'm in love with her." I couldn't believe what I was saying. I told Susan, "I'll have to talk to Maura about it."

The next person I told was Nancy, my weekday attendant. I thought she might want to quit on the spot or be uncomfortable undressing in front of me. I wasn't attracted to Nancy, and I didn't want her to feel like I had changed. I wasn't lusting after women. I just felt warm toward them, and comfortable and safe with them. Sometimes my fantasies unnerved me, and other times they felt quite natural. Nancy assured me I didn't have to worry about her leaving, and encouraged me to talk to Maura.

I spent a week trying to talk to Maura. I ended up staying

awake until one in the morning watching TV with her. During every commercial I vowed that during the next one I would tell her. Several times each night I would say good-night and go into the bedroom, only to return to the living room to try to tell her.

Thursday night, as I drifted in for the third time, she said, "Connie, are you sure nothing's wrong?"

"No, I just wanted to say goodnight again." I went back into the bedroom and tried to go to sleep. I was shaking with the fear of telling her, and the fear of not telling her. If I told her, that might mean I was a lesbian. If I told her I had sexual feelings for her, she might not feel the same and then I would have to deal with rejection. If I didn't tell her, I might lose her to this other woman whom I'd never met, but already disliked out of jealousy.

I developed a terrible chest cold which required that I begin to use the Intermittent Positive Pressure Breathing (IPPB) machine that I had used when I had the flu. The doctors insisted that I use it twice a day from that point on whether or not I had a cold. I began to notice that I coughed and wheezed a good deal more when Maura was around. I felt that the stress of keeping my secret from her was adding to my illness.

I wrote Maura a note, telling her that I couldn't talk about her leaving yet because it was upsetting me more than I understood and I didn't want to talk about it. I thought this might encourage her to ask me about it. As a woman, I had been taught that in order to get what I needed from someone I was attracted to, I should be indirect. Maura, on the other hand, had grown beyond her sexist training and was very direct. So when I said I didn't want to talk about it, she took me seriously and didn't bring it up.

When I got tired of waiting, wheezing and coughing, I went into the living room and said, "Maura, there's something I have to talk to you about that I can't talk to you about."

She said "Okay, Connie," and turned back to the television.

I went in my room and read for a while. Susan, the attendant, who was cleaning the refrigerator, whispered, "Tell her!"

I went back in and announced, "Maura, I'm having a lot of feelings about you that I don't understand and don't know what to do with. I don't expect you to feel the same way."

"I had gotten that impression from your note. It's all right. It'll take me a while to catch up with your feelings. A lot of times straight women have feelings about lesbians and lesbians have to be careful because they can get very hurt. It's hard to extend yourself and allow yourself to care about someone and then have the person several weeks or months later decide that they don't want to be with you because you're a woman. I'll have to think about it."

I breathed a sigh of relief. "That's fine. You don't have to think about it. I don't expect you to love me, or love me the same way, I just wanted you to know that I think you are wonderful and that I love you."

One night I invited all the women in my extended family for dinner. I didn't have enough room in my apartment to invite the men, and since I was learning so much about how women have things in common with each other that are different from what men want to talk about, I wanted there to be space for that.

Maura was supposed to go out that night, but she didn't. She wound up staying for dinner. I was pleasantly surprised. After everyone left I sat on the couch with her as I had done once in a while. We drank a glass of wine. We held hands. My heart was pounding. She said, "Well?"

I said, "Well what?"

"Well what do you think? How do you feel?"

"I told you how I feel. How do you feel?"

She started to giggle and put her arm around me. And we kissed. It was the most wonderful kiss in the whole world. We became very passionate. Maura rubbed me and I stroked her as best I could. I had my attendant put me in bed and leave us alone. Maura made love to me in the most special way that I had ever been made love to. Ron had touched my clitoris before but not very often. When Maura touched me there it felt like there was a whole world between my legs that went up inside of me and into every cell. She knew exactly what she was doing. She didn't hurt me. She asked me how I was after I came many times. I said wonderful. She said that sometimes women are frightened after the first time that they make love with another woman. I told her that I wasn't frightened at all, it was much better than the fantasies.

"Nancy, could you hand me the phone?" I put out my hand, propped up with my other hand for support. Nancy put the phone in my hand, and I gave her the number to dial. "Thanks," I whispered to Nancy. "Hi, Pidgie? How are you doing?"

"I'm okay. Are you going to the Muscular Dystrophy Association beach party tomorrow?"

"Yeah," I said. "But, there's something I want to tell you first."

"What's the matter?" she said nervously. "Are you sick?"

"No. But there's been something I've wanted to tell you for a while now, and I've been a little nervous about it. I've been involved with someone, kind of, but it's different."

"What do you mean?"

"Well . . . you know my roommate Maura? Well she and I have gotten kinda close, and . . . well she's a lesbian. I don't know if you knew that, but . . . Well, anyway, remember that night that you and Mommy and Carol and Aunt Kay and Aunt Ro and all the women were here?"

"Yeah, but what do you mean?" she pressed.

"Well, I mean that I'm involved with her. And I've never been so happy in my life. It feels natural, it feels normal, and I don't want you to freak out tomorrow, but I want to bring her to the beach party."

There was a long silence.

"Pidgie? Are you still there?"

"Yeah, I hear what you're saying."

"How do you feel about it?" I asked.

"I don't know. I mean, if you're happy, that's fine Conn. I know you had a lot of problems with Ron and a lot of stuff going on for you. And if this is what makes you happy . . . But I think I'm going to have to get used to it. Did you tell Mom?"

"No, and don't you either!"

"Are you kidding? I wouldn't dare! That's for you to do." She laughed. "What do you, like, do together, you know?"

"Well, physically it's not that much different from when I was with Ron. Only it's even better because Maura really understands me. Anyway, I'll make some potato salad and bring hamburgers tomorrow. Are you bringing anything?"

"Yeah. Hot dogs! Unless that's offensive to you," and she burst into laughter.

I laughed with her and it really broke the tension.

The next day, shortly before we all left the beach party, Pidgie pulled me aside, and said, "You look so good, Conn. I've never seen you this happy, and you know what? I'm not even freaked out or nervous. It just seems so natural with you two. But I don't know what you are going to do about Mom. I hope you're okay, and I hope everything goes well for you."

I decided that since my sister knew, I had to tell my brother. I called him up and invited him over for dinner. After dinner, as we were having dessert, I began, "So Frankie, how do you feel about gays?"

"What, those queers! I don't know . . ." He shuffled in his

seat. "I mean I had plenty of, you know, classmates and shit
at the Culinary Institute who were gay, and there were a
couple of dykes but, like, I wasn't really friends with them,
but they're okay. Why?"

"What would you say if I told you I was gay?" I looked
him dead in the eye.

"Jesus Christ, you got to be kidding! No!"

"Yeah, I've been in a relationship with a woman. I don't
know how you'll feel about it, but I wanted you to know."

"Oh Christ! Did you tell Ma?"

"No, and I don't want you to either."

"Don't worry man, no way." He moved back in his chair.

One night soon after, we went to a women's coffeehouse
in New York City. I overheard a conversation that Maura
had with one of the women there.

"Who's that woman you're with?" asked a woman in a
denim suit.

"Who, Connie? I live with her."

"You live with *her*? You don't have to live with her. I know
a lot of women looking for roommates. There's plenty of
lesbian space without women like that."

"Well, thank you, but I'm really okay where I am."

"Yes, but why should you live with someone like *that* . . . "

Their conversation was interrupted by a friend of Maura's
coming over and giving her a hug. Maura turned and introduced me as her "roommate." I felt the same shame of being
disabled that I often felt when Ron introduced me to his
other girlfriends. Maura had been quick to put Ron down for
choosing other able-bodied women over me, and even
though Maura wasn't doing that, she certainly didn't seem
proud of being lovers with me. I was angry at her for intro-
ducing me only as her "roommate," and I was angry at the
women I was meeting for their condescension and lack of
support.

I couldn't tell how much of Maura's and my problems were because of differences in our needs, or lack of support in handling our differences, but we were only lovers for a few weeks. Maura was having more and more difficulty with her back injury. Also, during lovemaking she needed a lot more pressure and movement than I could give, and for a longer time than I had stamina for. She was not comfortable with pleasuring herself with as much participation as I could manage.

Maura left, and I went through a long period of adjustment. I wasn't sure if I was a lesbian or not, or if I ever wanted to be in a relationship again with anyone. I went to the local women's bar for several months, but no one would talk to me. Several women at the bar asked my attendant why she brought her "patient" to this kind of place. My attendants explained that I was there because I was a lesbian and they were there because they were working for me.

I began writing poetry about my relationship with Maura and my joy at finding the depth of my love for women. I wrote about my body. I could barely move, yet felt so much pleasure at being touched. It was excruciating to be rejected for my body's imperfections and forced by others' assumptions to live as if I couldn't love. I knew I could love, and I wrote about it.

I entered a "gong" show at the lesbian bar. I read five of my erotic poems and won the hundred dollar prize. I felt I had won far more than a hundred dollars, though, because suddenly women were offering to buy me drinks and talking to me about where I lived and what I did. One of the women taught me to play Russian backgammon. Over the next few weeks I became the bar champion and beat everybody at the game. Through my poetry they were able to see me as a lesbian like them, and through my competing with them at games, they accepted me as one of the gang. At the bar I got to know more and more about women's culture. Although I had gained acceptance as one of the regulars, I was still not seen as someone to make love with.

I went to a local women's music event. There were lots of lesbian performers, including this big dyke named Maxine Feldman. She came out on stage in a formal tuxedo wearing red sneakers. I happened to have my red sneakers on too, and she spotted them from up on stage. "And there's another dyke with red sneakers! What's your name?"

I blushed. No one had ever acknowledged me as a dyke before. "Connie Panzarino," I shouted.

"Connie Panzarino! Hello, Connie Panzarino. It's nice to have you here." Maxine went into her comedy routine and sang some songs while I tried to be inconspicuous. I liked her attention, but I also felt shy.

I was asked to speak at a lesbian-feminist conference about what it was like to be disabled in the lesbian community. I met several other lesbians with disabilities there and we formed an organization. I began speaking at other conferences and classes, and I put together workshops about problems faced by people with disabilities. Things I'd thought and seen all my life started to come together, and I was able to articulate many concepts and causes of disability oppression.

I remember one particular workshop at Hunter College.

"It's like being fat. People reject me even though my body is healthier when I'm fat, and I'm happier when I'm fat. But people feel sorry for me, or they don't talk about food in front of me, or all they'll talk about is food in front of me. It makes me angry," the large, attractive woman in the blue dress challenged.

"I agree, except I get excluded because I'm small!" shouted a four-foot-tall woman in jeans, seated in the front row. "Nobody asks me out if they're going dancing. I'm fine to ask along to a movie, where it's dark, but people don't like being seen with me in public if it looks like I'm their date."

"There is an ancient taboo against people with disabilities being sexual or marrying," I explained. "Society used to protect itself from spreading disease by isolating people with illnesses, like in the leper colonies. In some states, even to-day, they still have antiquated laws forbidding people with epilepsy to marry. Even though we know better ways to control the spread of disease and most disabilities are not contagious, we are still, for the most part, isolated in institutions.

"Another unconscious, ancient reason for rejecting those of us with disabilities is related to the penal system of the old days. If a person stole something, he might get his arm chopped off. A missing limb or a deformity was thought to be the stigma of crime, and later, a sign of being a sinner. No *good* person would want to be seen with someone like that."

"Nothing's changed!" A man in a brown suit shifted in his wheelchair.

"I disagree," I responded. "Just us being in this room talking about it is a big change. And there is a whole movement out there for civil rights for people with disabilities now that didn't exist twenty years ago."

"I don't understand, then, why people stare at us if they don't want to see us." The man in the brown suit shifted again.

"People are often attracted to that which they are most afraid of," replied the woman in jeans, "that is why our first jobs were as freaks in the circus."

"But it's different now," pleaded the woman in the blue dress.

"I don't know if it's so different now," I replied. "When I work, I'm not considered disabled by law even though I can barely move, and when I'm not working, I'm often asked to speak at various places for honoraria, which is still money, to *educate* able-bodied people about what it's like to be disabled, or straight people about what it's like to be a lesbian. When I do that, I feel like I'm getting paid for being disabled. Of course, I suppose it's better than speaking for free, but sometimes I'm not so sure if it's any different from being in the sideshow, except that maybe I become the main at traction."

"You're right!" A man with a white cane and dark glasses exclaimed. "Nothing's changed much since the circus. It's so stupid. They act like they're exempt. I mean, anybody can become disabled. I didn't become blind until I was twenty-three."

"That's right! There is no such thing as an able-bodied person, really They're just temporarily able bodied." I smiled.

"TAB's!" giggled an Hispanic woman in a wheelchair.

The laughter was uplifting as it spread through the room. The validation and mutual respect was invigorating. We talked about how difficult it was to accept or adjust to a disability if you were able-bodied because disability was liter ally seen by many as a fate worse than death.

Eventually I learned, by teaching others and sharing experiences, that disability oppression was part of a larger oppression which many of us began to call ableism. Ableism seemed to be about using people's differences to create power imbalances which served those who created them. I continued exploring and defining how the fundamentals of sexism and racism might be based in ableism.

I started doing workshops on ableism. The workshops I did in the disabled community often dealt with sexism and homophobia. The workshops in the gay and lesbian community focussed on changing attitudes towards persons with disabilities. I challenged professionals who worked with disabled persons to come out of the disabled closet if they had a disability, and release us from the pedestalled prisons where they kept us. I realized one of the most effective ways I could change attitudes would be to work within their system, armed with credentials they'd respect. I decided to go back to school full time.

. . .

I was accepted into the New York University Art Therapy program. I was excited at the opportunity to study with Edith Kramer, who had developed art therapy when working with children from concentration camps in Eastern Europe. My court case, which Curtis Brewer of Untapped Resources was pursuing, was moving slowly. Federal and state legislatures were passing some parts of bills I had helped write.

That September I started at NYU and moved into the only accessible dormitory in Greenwich Village, but I still went back to my apartment on weekends. I got a roommate to help cover the apartment costs so I could still keep it while I was in school.

One night during my first year in school, while I was writing a paper on the development of sexuality, I noticed I was having difficulty writing. Within a few short weeks I could no longer move two of my fingers on my right hand. I had already lost most of the little use I had of my left hand over the last several years. Holding a pen or pencil to write or draw with became very difficult. It also took a great deal of effort to feed myself, so I began to use long-handled plastic ice cream spoons. They were lighter and I didn't have to lift my hand up so high in order to reach my mouth. I consulted with several different doctors and occupational therapists to see what could be done. Each one had a different opinion, but none had any viable solutions. Some thought it was a progression of my disability. Others said because of positioning and lack of muscle tone, the tendons were slipping off the knuckles. They could be repaired surgically if I didn't have a neuromuscular disease, but since I did, none of the surgeons would operate. They said I risked losing even more use of my hand if I had surgery.

I began wearing a splint in bed at night and used splinting devices to help hold my painting and drawing implements. I had to continue my art work in order to complete my Master's degree in art therapy. The Vocational Rehabilitation Commission provided a tape recorder and transcriber for my notes and papers. My attendants began to feed me more of the time to save my energy. I was told that if I didn't use my hand at all the muscles would atrophy, and if I pushed it to the point of fatigue I would lose use of it faster. No matter what I did, I was eventually going to lose use of my entire hand. I could no longer dial the phone or hold it independently.

This new level of dependence on others was terrifying. I cried and raged in my roommate's arms many days and nights. Her name was Michelle. We became close as I struggled to figure out new ways to cope and remain in school. Mary Ann, a close friend that I met in New York City, did movement massage with me and tried many natural remedies. I was having more and more difficulty with respiratory infections, in part from the emotional stress and in part from living in Manhattan with its air pollution.

I tried to learn more about my disability. I made appointments with the heads of rehabilitation in three of the leading university hospitals. One of them was the doctor I had seen as a child at the Institute. He insisted that I be admitted for a two-week evaluation because he hadn't seen me in so many years.

"What are you saying? What tests would you want to run and why? I'm relatively healthy and I just want more information about how this muscle disease might progress and why."

"Well, Connie darling, what can I tell you? I had a young woman like you, bright, a lot of drive, went to college, got married, got a job, and one night she just died."

I fought back the tears. "I'll get back to you." When I got home, I called Dr. Madonia. He was furious at the university doctor. He assured me that I was not in danger of dying in my sleep any time soon and said he would speak with the other doctor and have him justify all of the tests he intended doing over the two-week period. Dr. Madonia explained to me that most of the university hospitals are motivated more by research than by patient care.

The next day, Dr. Madonia called me back and said that the only tests that were justifiable were a chest X-ray and a pulmonary functions test to help the doctors determine if over the years my respiratory condition had worsened. Both of these tests could be done in one afternoon as an outpatient.

I saw a respiratory specialist, Dr. Alba, at another university hospital. She explained that my disease was much more related to post-polio syndrome than to the muscular dystrophies, because the problem was in the anterior horn cells of my spine. This meant that after twenty-eight and a half years of living with the disease, my nerve cells were beginning to die out and could not be replaced. She explained that this happens to post-polio patients as well, and that short periods of rest and avoidance of fatigue were the keys to continued functioning.

"Am I going to die? I mean, am I going to die sooner than the average person? *The Merck Manual* says my life expectancy is only two years, and most of my friends with dystrophy are dead, so I want to know the truth."

"Well, Connie," explained Dr. Alba, "there's no inherent reason why someone with your disability should not live a long life, as long as they don't get pneumonia that can't be cleared up, or choke to death. You see, the first swallowing muscle is a voluntary muscle, so it is affected by your condition. That's why you have difficulty swallowing."

"So other than choking on mucus, or getting pneumonia, I'm relatively safe?"

"Well, no, you could choke on food, too."

"I have often choked on food before. Would it help if I pureed my food in a blender, or ate baby food?"

"Yes, that's a very good idea. You would probably get better nutrition that way as well."

I thanked her and left, feeling angry that all these years

no one had ever suggested such a simple solution. I bought a blender and experimented with blending cafeteria foods in my dorm room. In spite of the losses I was experiencing, I felt I had gained power over my destiny. Instead of remaining a victim of the fear of dying, I could take steps to increase my chances of survival.

A few weeks later I received a letter from the Disabled Students Office informing me that the administration had to indefinitely put off installing wheelchair-accessible showers. "How the hell am I supposed to stay healthy if I can't stay clean?" I thought to myself.

Several of the disabled students had already fallen while trying to take showers or baths in the undersized, non-regulation tubs in our bathrooms. My Hoyer bathtub lift would not fit in these tubs.

"Nancy," I shouted. "Grab me some paper and a Magic Marker." I began to draw up a flyer appealing to the New York University student population to hold a shower strike to show their solidarity with the disabled students who could not shower. I showed a picture of a dirty looking person in a wheelchair, sweating, and saying "together we could raise a stench that would rock the administration into action." Nancy and I went to the copy machine and made five hundred copies. We put them all over New York University and Greenwich Village.

The next day, *The Village Voice* called and came over to take a photo and interview me and several other disabled students on the issue. My hair looked greasy, and I was proud of it. Less than a week after the paper came out, the university reversed their position and began constructing accessible showers in each accessible room in the dorm.

During that year, I formed a new organization called the Disabled Lesbian Alliance. We had eight members and met every other week for support and to plan political action.

We began to network nationally and ensured our visibility at lesbian and gay events. We encouraged other women with disabilities to come forward and participate, as well as to force more organizations to provide accessibility.

I decided to participate in the Gay Pride March in New York City. My brother unplugged all the TV sets in the house so my parents wouldn't see me on the news. I had to march by myself that day because my straight attendant said, "I support you in what you're doing, I just don't want to march with you because people will think I'm gay too. I understand why you're gay. After all, you're disabled and it's hard for you to find a man. It must be much easier for you to be a lesbian." I was dumbfounded by her "logic."

I asked my cousin Carol to work as my attendant the weekend of the march. She couldn't march with me because there would have been a major family feud if anyone had found out, but she met me every ten blocks on a corner to give me something to drink, and to see if I was all right. She met me at the end of the rally to help me go to the bathroom, but none of the port-a-johns were accessible. She and two of the other women helped me "go" into a paper cup behind the bushes. My hand was calloused from driving the chair the whole parade route and I looked a mess, but I was proud.

16

BEECHTREE

Sherri, one of the Disabled Lesbian Alliance members, said, "I think it would be great if some of us went to Michigan to the Women's Music Festival. I know it's camping and it's not very accessible, but there will be three thousand women there from all over the country. What an opportunity for us to help make change. Besides, it would be a blast!"

"I'd love to go," I said excitedly. "We could fit at least four or five of us in my van."

I had not been sexual with anyone since I was with Maura several years before. I went to the Michigan Women's Music Festival determined that I would find a lover, or at least make love with someone. On the way there, I wore dresses and skirts because it was easier to go to the bathroom on the eighteen hour ride if all I had to do was pull up my skirt and slide the bedpan under me. But because my skirt bunched up under me, when I got to Michigan my clitoris was broken open and bleeding. Women from the "Womb," the health care area, came over and put ointment on me and told me I should lie on my back with my legs open as much as possible, and keep it dry. There were several thousand women that year at Michigan, and I wanted to be sexual. How was I going to keep it dry? I was pretty upset.

I loved the festival. It was a safe environment where you

221

could walk in the woods at night and know that there were no rapists or muggers hiding. When it was hot out, you could take off your shirt. It was the first time I met so many other disabled lesbians. I saw many different kinds of bodies, and felt so much acceptance that it was only three days before I was zooming around in my chair in the sun wearing nothing but my red sneakers.

I ran a workshop on body image for women with disabilities. There were thirty women who attended, and I ran the workshop naked, not to be an exhibitionist, but because I felt comfortable. Some women came naked and others took off their clothes to show old scars from surgeries. We were angry about how our bodies had been looked at by doctors, by men, by family and by other lesbians. Women wept with grief at the pain and the shame they had endured. We held and rocked each other, and stroked each other's scars. Some of the scars reminded women of pictures of exotic dragons or beautiful flowers.

I felt good about my body, but was not able to be sexual because of the sore I had developed. On the last night of the festival, I was lying down in my van feeling depressed about not having met a lover. I debated whether or not to go down to the night stage for the last concert. Some of the women I had met at the festival came by and asked me to go sit with them. While we were on our way to the concert area, a red-haired woman chased me down the hill, shouting, "I'm in love with you! I've read all about you and saw your picture in JEB's book. I've been going to all your workshops hoping to talk with you, but I chickened out, and I just can't leave Michigan without telling you that I love you and that I want to be with you."

I stopped and smiled. "Why don't you come and sit down with me at the concert? Maybe we can talk." I thought to myself, "This must be some kind of joke." I had been praying to the goddess about finding a lover here, but this was a little bit much. She sat down on the ground and leaned against my chair. "What's your name?" I asked.

"Kaicha," she replied.

"Where are you from?"

"Oregon."

"Well, I'm from New York." I breathed a sigh of relief because I would probably never see her again.

She smiled, "I know, I'm coming to New York to be with you."

I panicked, but continued talking. My sore clitoris began to hurt. I must be getting excited in spite of myself, I thought.

We went for a walk to one of the bonfires and sat for a while talking. "Where did you get the name 'Kaicha'?" I asked. "It's unusual."

"I got it in a Native American circle. It means New Beginnings."

She put her arm around me and was about to kiss me just as a flash of lightning hit very close. It started to rain, and we had to run back to my van. We fumbled with the lift in the dark and the rain. When we got in my van, I asked my two attendants to leave us alone for a while. They went off, draped in ponchos. Once again Kaicha leaned forward to kiss me. Just then two friends, Kady and Pagan, opened the van and pushed in our blind friend, Marge, saying, "Connie, we're gonna leave Marge here for a little while until the storm clears. We'll be right back." Marge couldn't see that I was with someone. I turned red with embarrassment, not only because I was with someone but because it seemed awful for Marge to have been thrust into someone's space and left there just because she was blind.

After a few seconds of silence, I said, "This is Kaicha. She and I are spending some time in the van." We talked small talk at first, then Marge told me all about the Women's Braille Press which was taping radical lesbian feminist books for blind women, and women like me who couldn't turn pages to read by themselves. After the rain stopped Kady and Pagan came and got Marge. My attendants came back at the same time.

Kaicha said, "I'd better go, I have to check on my son at the boys' camp before the last shuttle. I'll be back in the morning to see you off. I'll need your address so I can come see you next week. I'm coming to New York, and I know you don't believe me, but I am."

She was right, I didn't believe a word of it.

Kaicha did come to New York about two days after we got back.

"Do you like lasagna?" I looked up at Kaicha. "I made lasagna."

"Sounds great!"

After dinner, I asked her what she'd like to do that evening.

She said, "I'd like to make love with you."

I thought to myself, "That was direct." To her I said "All right," and we went to bed. We didn't actually make love that first night, although we did touch a lot and talk intimately. The next day we went to the beach and I sat on her lap in the water. The water ebbed and flowed around us. We made love in the water.

Kaicha had another lover who was very warm and supportive of her relationship with me. During this time, I began to be lovers with my friend and attendant Michelle, with Mary Ann, and a friend named Janet. After nearly three years of being single, I was now enjoying several full relationships at the same time. Perhaps Ron was right. It was possible, and pleasant, to love more than one person at the same time and love them all equally, differently, and still have it work.

One afternoon, Dorothy, my transcriber for school, was dropping off my notes for me at NYU. She told me about a big farm house that was for sale across from where Kady and

Pagan lived, in Monticello, New York. She said that Barbara
Deming owned it and was trying to sell it to lesbians.

Barbara Deming was a lesbian feminist pacifist writer who
wrote many books and essays while living at her farm before
she became severely disabled in a car accident. Her body
couldn't tolerate the long, cold winters of upstate New York
any longer, so she had to move to Florida. She loved the
farm so much, she wanted to sell it to just the right person.

"Does it have a fireplace?" I asked Dorothy.

"I think so," she said.

"I'll buy it!"

"Panzarino, are you crazy? What are you saying?" asked
Nancy, my attendant.

"I probably am, but maybe not. After being at the festival
in Michigan and doing all the work I've been doing on ableism, I think there's a real need to create a space where disabled lesbians can live free from homophobia and ableism,
and be out where there's clean air to breathe, and good
healthy homegrown food to eat. I know I sound romantic,
but why not?"

When I got back to the apartment that weekend, Michelle and I talked about the possibility of moving there
while I was still in school. Michelle felt she could work on
her silversmithing just as easily from the farm as from our
apartment. We went up to see it and fell in love with it.
There were twenty-one acres of woods and fields. It had an
eight-bedroom farmhouse that had only one step so it was
easily rampable. There were also outbuildings and a well.

Kady decided she wanted us as neighbors, so she wrote to
Barbara Deming. Several days later, Barbara called to offer
me a mortgage, with financial terms I couldn't refuse, under
the condition that I would be up there within two weeks. I
had wanted Michelle to be partners in purchasing the land,
but Michelle felt that she was not ready to make a commitment. Barbara also did not want to have to keep changing
her agreement to suit others, so she and I decided that the

mortgage would be my sole responsibility. I was to be, as Kady called it, a "landlordess." I was thirty-two years old.

As Michelle and I began packing we shouted back and forth across the apartment. "We can grow corn!" I shouted.

"I can have a puppy!" exclaimed Michelle.

"Tomatoes!" I yelled.

"We can grow tofu!" she laughed.

"The cats will love it!" I squealed.

"I can have a bear cub!" said Michelle.

Michelle and I talked about how our parents were going to react to our moving to a farmhouse that would hopefully be filled with many lesbians. I had already "come out" to my mother on the phone one day because she had been asking questions about where my attendants slept in my apartment and why I only had pictures of women on my walls. I was afraid one of my lesbian friends might come up to me and give me a kiss while my parents and I were visiting in Greenwich Village, and that my mother would freak out. She had always warned me about lesbians and seemed to be really good at picking them out in a crowd. I remember being places with her when I was younger and hearing her whisper, "See that lady over there? She's queer."

My mother had been angry when I told her I was a lesbian. She said she would never suspect that of me, and she refused to believe it. She said some people were born that way and couldn't help it, but I had a choice. If I was choosing that kind of lifestyle, according to her, I was a sick person. She told me not to tell my father or anyone else. I agreed not to tell my father, but said I had already told my brother and sister and my relatives. So then she was angry because she felt she was the last to know. But as time went on, she tried to accept me and my sexuality as much as she could.

Now I felt that since I was moving to a household where my sexual orientation would be more obvious, I had a responsibility to tell my father. I wrote him a letter. When my aunts and uncles found out that I had written him, they became furious and intercepted the letter before he found it. They tried to protect him as if he were a child. My uncle and my mother said he would die of a heart attack—even though his heart was fine. I got very angry and I told them that I would call my father myself, and tell him that they had the letter if they didn't give it to him.

When my father read the letter, he did get angry at me, but he didn't die. I didn't know how much of the anger was really his, or how much of it was my mother's because she expected him to be furious. My father didn't speak to me. He forbade me to see my sister because I might "influence" her. I saw her anyway. In fact, my sister showed up at my dorm with my father's van, unbeknownst to him, and helped me move to the farm.

We had a good time driving up to the farm. Pidgie and I talked back and forth on the CB radios.

"Hi, Conn? It's beautiful up here. Over."

"This is the Blueberry Express," I said, using my CB handle. "Wait till you see the farm, you're going to flip out!"

"Conn, you're supposed to say 'over' when you're done at the end. Over."

"Okay! Over." We drove along further and further into the hills, leaving the city behind us. All of a sudden, the radio crackled. "Conn! Conn! Are you there? Over."

"Quick, grab the CB," I shouted to my attendant. "My sister's in trouble!" My attendant held the mike with one hand as she steered with the other, and pressed the button on the mike. "Pidgie! Are you okay? Over."

"Conn! We just passed the exit that Harry lives off of. That's where I lost my virginity. Right there!"

"Pidgie, I think we should wait and talk about this later. I thought something happened to you. I want to relax for a while. I'm tired. I'll talk to you when we get there, unless you have a problem. Okay? Over."

"Sure, Conn. But I just wanted to tell you that it was great! Over."

We had to get upstate fast and unpack the van so she could get back down to the city before my dad knew she was gone. As soon as we arrived on the land, my sister and I took off for the far field together. Kaicha told me later she had tears in her eyes watching the two of us bouncing over the land, side-by-side in our wheelchairs. We watched the sunset together.

"I can't believe it, Conn! It's so beautiful. You know, I never told you this, but I never thought you would live this long. And I guess I didn't know what that meant for me. Do you get scared sometimes?"

I sighed. "Yeah, a lot. I think I'll be healthier here. And you can come up whenever you want. I'm really grateful that you came up here to help me move today. I mean, this is the first time that you've put your neck out for me no matter what Mom and Dad might think or say."

"Yeah, well I'm twenty-one now. I can do what I want. Besides, I think they're being stupid about this. I mean you're not any different than you used to be. Besides, what are sisters for!" Pidgie reached out and touched my hand. "You know we can never even hug like regular sisters."

"I know. Sometimes I felt like I didn't want to touch you. I think because I couldn't hug you, or hold you, like I could hold Frankie, it got really mixed up for me. I also think sometimes I was really mean to you because I didn't like myself very much. I want you to know, I'm really sorry." My eyes filled up with tears.

"Conn, stop. You're going to make me cry. I didn't treat you so hot either." For the first time in our lives, Pidgie and I told each other we loved each other.

A few weeks later, Kaicha went back to Oregon. I remember smiling and sobbing as she pulled out of the driveway. I asked my attendant to pick up my hand and wave it for me.

Kaicha was waving, crying, and driving all at the same time. I turned and looked to my friend Kady for comfort.

"Ain't worth spending time with 'em if you can't cry over 'em when they leave." Kady took a long, hard puff on her cigarette and blew the smoke upwards defiantly. Kaicha and I maintained our relationship long distance, and spent time together every few years.

I named the land and house Beechtree, after the huge double beech tree that Barbara Deming and I both loved so much. The air was wonderful there. I became much healthier without breathing the city's air pollution, even though it was very cold in the winter. Michelle made a sled for me with a chair-back nailed onto it so I wouldn't have to be housebound when the snow came. The other women in the house could pull me in the snow. Even when it was too cold to go out, the gorgeous view from each window was enough to keep our spirits high. I learned to bake, both for fun and to keep the kitchen warm.

Each of the women at the farm was committed to confronting her own ableism. As a group we were to try to eliminate ableism in our living space, our working lives, and in the world at large. Several of the women who stayed at Beechtree had epilepsy. When they started to feel that they had a seizure coming on, they got down on the floor so as not to fall down. Sometimes it passed, and they didn't have a seizure. Some of us needed to lie down for other reasons, so we decided that each room would have either a daybed or a couch or at least a mat on the floor. Lying down became a norm, and even some of the more able-bodied women used the couches just to rest.

Abby, one of the big, strong women who lived there, had a bad back. In the fall when she was going to put up the storm windows, Maggie offered, "Hey Ab, if your back seems to get tired let me know, okay? I'll be glad to help."

Abby just nodded. It was up to her to decide what was too much and what wasn't. It was helpful for other women to check in with her during the day to see if she needed a hand, but confronting ableism was not about taking control for someone or setting that person's limits.

For example, one day when I was out walking with Liza, I noticed that she began to move a little slower and her breathing became heavier. I said, "Liza, do you need some support to take a break right now? You look like you're getting tired."

"No. I'm okay."

I accepted that Liza knew what she needed and had the right to refuse and figure out what to ask for. It was always up to the individual woman to decide if she needed to rest; and it was all right for any woman to ask others to intervene for her if she knew she had difficulty knowing when to stop.

One day Michelle came into the kitchen and said, "Panzarino, I need to talk to you about something."

"Sure." I turned my chair and started to roll into the living room.

"No, not in there. I need to talk to you in my room."

I nodded assent, and she picked me up and carried me up three flights of stairs to her room. She sat me in a chair near her bed and we talked. She had initiated the conversation, and wanted it to be private, and I knew that if she had wanted to talk to Suki, Maggie or Abby alone she would have asked them to her room, so she was just trying to make it an equal situation for me. Michelle was very special in that way. She often asked me to go for walks in weather that neither my sled nor my wheelchair could accommodate; she would carry me out to a field, and sit me on her lap or on a stone fence where we talked and watched the dogs playing.

Equity was an important theme at Beechtree. We strove to make our lives work without the power imbalances so ingrained in us by our patriarchal society. One day Kady and Pagan sent a note to the women at Beechtree asking them to help cut wood. The note was addressed to everyone but me. The Beechtree women all refused to help unless they asked me as well. It was up to me to choose to refuse. If I couldn't do the task, I might be able to do it with the help of my attendant, or to work out an exchange with another woman in the area to do part of my share of the work if I did something for her in exchange. Kady and Pagan never failed to include me in their asking of favors again. Liza, a woman with Crohn's disease, was having a severe exacerbation at one point and could not even get out of bed. We had all decided to go pick wild flowers. When we got back, Maggie and I collected all the vases in the house, filled them with water, and brought them to Liza's bedside along with the flowers. Her job was to help us arrange them in the different vases. That way she took part in the activity. She loved it!

Living at Beechtree was about not just accepting disability or difference, but celebrating it. It was easy to honor difference when one lived so close to nature and saw so much diversity. It became easier as we learned how valuable each of our differences and differing perspectives were.

Each season brought its own delights. The spring brought luscious mud from melting snows, fawns cavorting with their mothers, and new growth everywhere. It meant lots of work in the garden—work that continued through the summer.

I learned to plant, grow and harvest most of our food. I volunteered to take responsibility for the seedlings. I felt that was something I could do easily indoors, and I was raring to go on this garden thing anyway. This didn't mean that I would not participate in the actual planting, pulling weeds or harvesting, but each of us took responsibility for different aspects of the garden. Maggie took charge of the actual planting since she had the most experience with that. My seedlings thrived until I had to thin them. I could not bear to pull our the straggling, smaller, slightly deformed seedlings and let the healthier ones grow. Instead, I pulled out all the healthy ones. The seedlings looked pathetic, and the women in the house were upset for fear that none of them would grow. To all of our amazement, we had very healthy plants that year. The small little "disabled" seedlings grew strong and were able to survive the abundance of rain we had that year followed by intense heat.

I learned to leave spider webs in the house to catch the flies and mosquitoes. I studied feminism with Kady, Pagan and other women passing through, and got in touch with Mother Nature, and the goddess within myself. I read of the destruction of female worship and images of the goddess by the Catholic Church centuries ago. I saw this as part of male domination and Christian patriarchal religion. I began to see how organized religion oppressed and enslaved women throughout the world. Besides, they didn't let disabled women be nuns.

I had been a devout Catholic, and then became a liberal Christian. The Bible students that I studied with were wonderful to me. They didn't judge me. They helped me get settled in California. They helped me build ramps. They helped me understand that much of the Bible had been misinterpreted and turned into lies that would serve the political times. What they didn't see was that they also were still misinterpreting a lot of the Bible. For instance, in the Old Testament the Bible refers to men having sex with men as sinful because they're wasting seed. In this day and age when we are choosing birth control and abortion because there are too many children, the wasting of seed would not be a sin. In addition, the Bible does not speak about women loving women as a sin because that did not affect the population. Women often loved women in harems. And, when the various patriarchs mentioned in the Bible had more than one wife, those women loved each other and often expressed it physically. I felt at peace with God as a Goddess also because I had learned through the Bible students that one of the words for God was a feminine word meaning the breasted one. This meant that God was neither a man nor a woman but probably both.

I could not bring myself to continue to attend Bible study classes because I knew that some of the brethren would be hurt by my being a lesbian. I also could no longer support the division between men and women within the Bible study classes. Men were supposed to speak and teach at conventions and conferences and in church on Sundays. The women, on the other hand, were there to comfort, cook organize and teach the children.

I knew that the Being that created this land was a loving, kind, all accepting One. And so I learned to love myself and to bless the bats that flew overhead at dusk and ate mosquitoes. I had lessons in neighborliness from the skunk that came into our kitchen at night through the cat door but who never sprayed inside our house. I learned to plant and identify herbs, which I began to use to strengthen my immune system, so I got sick less often.

Although my family never approved of my sexuality, they learned to appreciate that it was making me healthier and certainly happier. One Sunday in the summer, my whole family, including aunts and uncles and cousins, came up for a big barbeque. It rained all day, so my Dad put a large tarp in the branches of the double beech tree. We all ate under it and sang songs and went for walks in the rain.

My cousin, Gloria, came to see me at the farm with her partner, Barbara. She was still the beautiful strong woman I remembered from my childhood. She was proud of me, my lifestyle, and all that I had accomplished. Her approval more than made up for my family's less positive reaction.

Every fall brought living paintings all around me as the fields and woods changed every day. We harvested and stored as much produce as we could for the winters. We were busy for months preparing the house for the long season.

• • •

My body had changed somewhat for the better. Being on the land and breathing good air seemed to help. I had fewer respiratory infections and even fewer colds. This amazed me since the winter was so much more severe in Monticello than on Long Island. I was eating healthy foods and was surrounded by loving hands. I could no longer use my own hands at all. Whereas before, I was able to partially feed myself, now I had to be totally fed. It was as if the silverware had gained a pound a day until now it weighed five hundred pounds. I could not hold the phone. My parents bought me a headset for my telephone so I would be able to talk in private without having to have someone stand next to me and hold the phone. I began looking into assistive technology. It was difficult in a rural area to get information on puff-and-sip computers and other devices. I decided to go to the Rehabilitation Center for two weeks to be rehabilitated. The new name for my disability was now Werdnig-Hoffman's Disease, Type II. I had realized that since I had been born with a disability, I had never really been rehabilitated, just evaluated and studied.

At the Burke Rehabilitation Center I was fitted with devices which enabled me to feed myself. They showed me computers I could run, and environmental controls with which I could turn on televisions, radios, lights and door openers. They fitted me for an electric wheelchair with puff-and-sip control. A puff-and-sip switch is an on/off switch operated by breath control. By putting my lips around a little tube, I could puff or sip to operate numerous devices, or turn my chair in any direction. The staff opened up a world of possibilities for me, and then they discharged me. They said I would have to find funding for these things. I asked them where to look. They said that the wheelchair might be able to be paid by Medicaid and Medicare, but they didn't know how I could get the computer or the environmental control system. I started working through Vocational Rehabilitation to get a computer. I asked about the feeding devices. They said that those were not for sale. They were only available for use in the hospital. I was so angry.

In many ways, the two weeks there had been hell. There had been no full length mirror anywhere on the floor because the staff said, "We don't feel it's good for people to look at themselves. It's too much of a shock." Each morning I had had to race down to the elevator half dressed, take it one floor down, and finish dressing in front of the one mirror in the physical therapy department. It had been depressing to be there. Everyone there was unhappy about being disabled. I wasn't angry about being disabled, I was angry about not being able to get what was available to make me able to function better with my disability.

I came back home and talked to the other women on the farm about my losses. Since I could no longer use my hands, I could no longer feed myself, rub my eyes, pick my nose, spit into a tissue, scratch my head, hold the phone, do my art, touch my lovers or slap mosquitoes as they bit my face. I had a lot of grieving to do before I could learn to compensate for what I couldn't do. Eventually, I learned to direct my attendant more. I learned to use my eyes to point since I could no longer point with my hands. My cat, Dianna, was used to me petting her. Now she would put her head under my hand, crawl under it and let my hand slide down her body. My housemates learned to read books with me so they could sit next to me and turn pages. I realized that this was probably only the beginning of change for me. It was hard. Sometimes I was angry, other times I was scared. Mostly I was grateful to be in one of the most beautiful places on earth surrounded by supportive and loving women.

It was hard for me to be an active sexual partner. I learned to use my mouth, my breath and my creative voice to accompany my lovers in touching themselves. I painted many pictures in my mind, and knitted and embroidered in my dreams.

I went to see Edith Kramer and asked her to help me to learn to use my mouth for art. We started off small, doing circles and scribbles the way you do when you're a child. After a few hours I was able to draw people. After a few weeks I could sign my name with a pen in my mouth, and the signature exactly matched the signature from my hand. Handwriting is a frame of mind, I guess, and maybe it really does reflect one's personality.

I researched more about my disability. There was little to find. I conferred with Dr. Frank Karle, a wonderful chiropractor, with Susan Weed, an herbalist, and several massage therapists. I had had migraines and a continuous headache for several years. In three months, Dr. Karle eliminated my headaches. Following Dr. Alba's suggestion of pureeing my foods in a blender helped with my nutrition. I started with smoothies of fruit and yogurt, and then added nut butters. I soon began to realize that you can create deliciously nutritious meals by pureeing just about everything, including stir-fried foods and rice, in a blender. The food didn't look the same, but I looked better and better the more I ate pureed foods. Occasionally we went out to dinner, and I would bring my blender. People in restaurants seemed to have a hard time with it. I guess they were not used to preparing a beautiful plate of food and then have somebody blend it up. But I liked it. I even blended lobster on my birthday!

There were many women who came and went on the farm. All were lesbian or bisexual. Most were artists; some were disabled. Some came for a week, some for a month, some for several years. All were committed to fighting disability oppression. Sometimes that meant helping one another physically or emotionally, sometimes that meant letting a woman find her limits no matter how painful it was to watch, sometimes it meant reminding one another that we were different and could add different talents to Beechtree as a whole. Each woman was encouraged to do the chores that she liked to do the most and that were easiest for her. Sometimes the commitment meant admitting discomfort about disability.

Fighting oppression can create a supportive environment, but sometimes it is fraught with struggle. Whenever there were times of struggle, or when women left, it was very difficult for me. I often thought I had failed to create a supportive place. Once I went to the far field and meditated and asked the Goddess, "Why do the women leave? Why don't they stay?" The answer came that I was to stay, and that many women would come and go. Some would return often, but I was the permanent one to ensure that Beechtree would always exist.

I met a woman named Rebecca at the first Disabled Lesbian Conference which I organized with several other women. It was held in Michigan on the grounds of the Women's Music Festival in 1981 after the close of the festival. Rebecca had epilepsy. She was a therapist also, and won my heart and soul. She moved to the farm and became a strong force in many of my political struggles and in managing Beechtree.

Ron came to see me for a couple of days. He stayed in a motel near the raceway. We had nice walks on the land in our chairs, and a good long talk lying under the beech tree. Ron talked with Rebecca and the other women, and played with Dianna. A lot of his anger seemed to have passed. I was relieved to find that we could sit together as friends.

Some women came to visit from the Seneca Women's Encampment for the Future of Peace and Justice at the Seneca Army Depot in Romulus, New York. The peace camp was established to try to stop the U.S. from sending Pershing and Cruise missiles to Europe. They told us that the encampment was not accessible to women in wheelchairs. I went to the encampment with Shelly, my attendant, to conduct workshops on ableism and to get funding to build ramps and boardwalks to make the camp accessible. Kady organized a crew of women to do the actual building of the ramps.

When I came home, I was interviewed by the town newspaper. The next day I appeared in an article about the encampment. That afternoon, the county Medicaid office called to tell me that my attendants, who were being paid by them, would no longer be allowed to drive me outside the county. It was obvious to me that the conservative officials in the county had decided that I should not be involved in such radical political work as the Seneca Women's Encampment. One of the clerks at the checkout at the grocery store had made a comment to me that the taxpayers should not be paying people to help me organize against the government. I explained to her that I was not organizing against the government, I was organizing to insure that there would be life on the planet. Over the next several months, the county became more and more restrictive about who I could hire, and how much they could work. It became increasingly difficult to find attendants. Other women with disabilities who lived in the household tried to help me with my daily care when there were no attendants for several hours, or for overnights, but it was too difficult. Without attendants, I could not function. Without attendants to drive me, I could not look for work.

I put up posters and flyers in all of the local drugstores and at the local hospital calling for a meeting of people with disabilities who were having difficulties with transportation, employment, medical care, attendants, and so on. Fifteen people came to the first meeting. We formed an advocacy group and I began a lawsuit to contest the county's restrictions as a violation of my constitutional right to travel. The more I organized and fought back, the tighter they made the restrictions. The Upjohn Home Health Aide Agency, which was paid by the county to provide my attendants, told the attendants they had to keep written progress notes on my activities, including how often I brushed my teeth and how often I used the phone.

I had continued writing letters and articles on disability, feminism, sexuality and lesbianism. I decided it was time to write a book. I recorded sixteen hours of tapes in one weekend and six months later I taped another twelve hours. My intention was to hire people or find friends who would transcribe a draft so that I could eventually publish my story. It was hard at first to learn to write by dictating, even though I had done some dictation when I lost the use of my hands and could no longer write my case notes while attending New York University. I would visualize the words in my mind and then read them off the imaginary page onto the tape.

I finished my Master's degree in art therapy. I wrote my thesis in five days. It was easy after taping so much of the book. By then, I was allowed by law to work and still receive Medicaid benefits under a new SSI plan for achieving self-support (PASS) written by my attorney in New York. However, with the restrictions placed on me by the county, I could not find work that I could maintain. I did have a few private art therapy clients, but because I lived nine miles out of town and there was no public transportation, I could not develop a private practice that would bring in enough income to live on. I also continued to work part time at the Bennett Residence, an intermediate care facility in Liberty, New York developing an art therapy program for adults with developmental disabilities. Most of the residents were severely mentally retarded, and some had physical disabilities as well. They taught me a new level of interdependence. For example, a resident who was too "retarded" to speak would feed a resident who could not feed himself. Residents who could walk pushed those in wheelchairs who could not push themselves, and they in turn often spoke for residents who could not speak. I related better to the residents than to many of the staff. The residents accepted me in my wheelchair, and I was able to work with them in ways the other staff could not. I never used food as positive reinforcement. The art was reinforcement in itself. The money I earned at the ICF was enough to help pay my taxes, but not enough to pay my other expenses. I began to fall behind on my mortgage payments. Barbara Deming, from whom I had bought the farm, became ill with cancer. She called to say goodbye two weeks before she died. After her death, her verbal mortgage agreement with me was not honored by her executors, who were legally correct in their interpretation of the written mortgage agreement she and I had both naively signed. I began falling heavily in debt.

After five years of living on the farm, I faced losing the land and losing my dream. The house was home to me as no house had ever been, and each tree felt like a beloved friend.

17

BACK TO WORK

More and more of the women who lived at the farm were leaving to go to school or to join larger lesbian communities elsewhere. Because of the Medicaid attendant care problems I was encountering, women with similar disabilities who were considering moving to the farm felt discouraged. I was getting deeper into debt and more desperate since I still could not hire aides, and still had not won my right to travel outside Sullivan county. Rebecca had left shortly after we ended our three-and-a-half-year relationship. Our changing disabilities and the isolation and difficulties of the farm had become too much for her. After she left, living at the farm felt even more difficult since there was no one to share the emotional or financial burden. I decided to go to the Michigan Women's Music Festival again to network with other women who owned land and with other women with disabilities.

"Going down to the crafts area?" Ramona signed to me in ASL (American Sign Language). Her brown chest was gleaming in the sun, displaying strands of new-bought beads.

I nodded my head and smiled. "No money. Just looking." I looked to Susan, her friend, to interpret.

Ramona sighed, and nodded. She patted my shoulder and signed, "I understand. Times are hard." She waved and went on.

I drove my chair through the crafts area, not looking at anything. It was as if I was being drawn through the crowd by some force. I found myself a few minutes later in front of a display of stones and crystals. My eyes were fixed on the most beautiful smoky quartz crystal I had ever seen.

"How much is that one?" I said, pointing with my eyes. I held my breath as the craftswoman handed it to me. She put it in my lap, since I could not lift my hands to receive it.

"It's one hundred and twenty dollars." The craftswoman beamed at me. "It's a very special crystal. It will change your life. It makes wishes come true."

"It certainly will change my life," I thought to myself, "It'll make me poorer than I am." To her, I smiled and said, "No, thank you. I don't think I can afford it now."

I left the crafts area and went back to find my attendant, Kay, in the Disabled Area Resource Tent, which we called "DART." I felt pains in my chest similar to those I felt when Rebecca broke up with me. It felt like I had left something behind. I took my attendant with me back to the crafts area, back to the crystal. She helped me hold it in my hands for a while. I found myself smiling and weeping. I gave the crystal back, feeling much better, and went to eat dinner.

All through dinner, I kept feeling like there was a piece of me missing. I kept seeing that beautiful crystal. I knew I had to finish eating and get dressed warmly for the concert that evening. I had no time to spare, but I told my attendant to clean up the supper dishes and get herself ready and I would be right back. I drove my chair at top speed down to the crafts area just as the craftswomen were packing up for the night. I wove in and out of people and tables being broken down, and boxes being moved, straight to that powerful crystal.

"Would you consider taking a post-dated check for September first, when my disability check comes in?" I smiled and opened my eyes wide, the way I had learned to do on the Telethon. It was still just early August, so this was a long shot.

"Of course! I think that crystal has found its home." The craftswoman handed me the crystal and helped me get out my checkbook and write the check.

I flew back to the van, where we were camped, as fast as my chair could go. As I drove my chair, my mind wandered. For the first time since my break-up with Rebecca, I was thinking about how nice it would be to be close to someone again. I was glad I had met Linda, a sweet woman from Chicago who had multiple sclerosis and was also becoming deaf, and Diane Stein, a brilliant spiritual writer who was severely learning disabled. I also met several able-bodied women at the festival who were warm and affectionate. I knew I wasn't ready to have another lover, but I felt more open to feeling good than I had in a long time. I thought about the farm and whether or not I really wanted to go back there, because it was so hard. Before I knew it, I was back at the van.

"Quick, Kay, help me get dressed. My friend, Linda, is supposed to be here in half an hour to go to the last concert with us. Put me on the bed in the van and let me use the bedpan."

I lay on the bed, naked and clean after a sponge bath. Kay was about to help me put on my shirt when I got goosebumps and a tingling feeling all over. My body was responding quite pleasurably to something I had not even seen yet. I heard a sweet clear voice from the back of the van calling me by name. My heart started beating faster.

"Connie Panzarino?" The voice came again.

"Yes?" I answered.

"My name is Judy. Do you know Jeanne Freebody? Jeanne

is a friend of mine and said that you have an ex-lover with a disability that sounds similar to mine. Jeanne's been telling me to come over and talk to you."

I asked my attendant to turn my head so I could see out the back of the van. My eyes turned to an attractive, brown-haired dyke with big beautiful eyes that triggered the same physical response in my body that I had experienced a minute before. "Can you hang out for a few minutes?" I said. "I'm going to get dressed, and I'll be right out."

"Kay, hurry up! I have to get out there quickly," I whispered.

When I got out of the van, Judy and I talked for a few minutes. I invited her to come down to the concert and join Linda and me later on, which she did. I encouraged her to lean against my legs for back support while we watched the performance. I liked feeling her warm body against mine. My body seemed to know her, and my mind certainly wanted to.

That night I slept with my crystal in my hand. I dreamt about being able to stay at the festival all year-round.

The next day I bumped into Judy several times as she and I and the rest of the camp were packing up to leave. We hugged goodbye at every opportunity. Judy had signed a card with a message and her phone number for my old lover and friend, Michelle. I kept hoping that Judy would offer to take my number, but I felt too shy to ask for hers. I didn't know if it was appropriate to take her number off the card, so I was relieved when she mentioned that if I wanted to be in touch, she had left her phone number on the card and I was welcome to use it.

Several weeks after the Michigan festival I was to coordinate disabled services for the Northeast Women's Music Retreat. Two of my festival workers became ill a week before the festival. I thought about asking Judy to fill in for one of the workshifts. I really wanted her to come, but I left it up to fate and asked Linda instead. I figured if Linda couldn't come, then I would ask Judy. I tried to hide my joy when Linda said she couldn't make it. Then I called Bonnie, my assistant coordinator, who happened to live in Boston, and told her all about Judy.

"Well! Go ahead and ask her." Bonnie chuckled. "Tell her I'll give her a ride to the festival. She sounds great! Maybe she'll get you to move to Boston. We could sure use you up here. *Nothing's* accessible up here."

I sat back, took a deep breath, and envisioned how it all might work out. I knew enough about Judy's physical needs to do some planning. She had to eat every two hours, but I had already arranged for two refrigerators in Helen's Space, which was the area for women with disabilities, named for Helen Keller. I knew Judy had to lie down a good deal of the time, so I figured I could assign her the bunk by the door of the cabin porch, so she could even lie down on her shift if she needed to. I wanted her to come so badly that I was willing to do anything to make it possible. If she said no, she didn't want to come, I wanted it to be because she didn't want to, not because she couldn't.

That afternoon I called Judy. She seemed happy that I called, but told me she absolutely would not attend another festival that year, since she had had to spend most of the Michigan festival laying or crawling on the ground with fatigue. Then I asked her what would be hard about it. For every problem she told me, I told her how we could work it out. She seemed a little overwhelmed at my numerous accommodations, but she said she would think about it and get back to me.

Several days later Judy called to say she had found three women who would drive her car in exchange for rides to the festival. She said she could be at the festival that Friday eve-

ning. While I was happy, I was so busy at that point getting
ready for the festival that I wasn't as excited as I'd expected
to be.

When Judy arrived, we kissed hello and my heart started
pounding so fast I had to excuse myself. I went to see how
the disabled seating arrangements were down at the concert.
When I came back, we sat and listened to some music tapes I
had brought. I gave her a poem I wrote. In between welcom-
ing festi-goers, keeping track of my workers, and registering
women with disabilities, I spent time with Judy.

That night I lay in my van, wide awake, attempting to figure out the midpoint between Boston and Monticello. I
wished I was able-bodied, just so I could get up quietly,
without waking my attendant, get dressed, and figure out
some excuse for needing to go over to the cabin to check on
the refrigerators or something in case Judy might be up having another meal. We could hang out together, and I could
go back to bed, and no one would ever know.

The next morning I made a bee-line for the cabin as soon
as I got up. "Hi, Judy. How'd you sleep?"

"I couldn't sleep very well." Judy looked a bit pensive,
then smiled a smile that seemed incongruous for one who
hadn't slept all night. "How about you?"

"I didn't sleep very well either." I hesitated a minute.
"How come you didn't sleep well?"

She turned a bit red. "Well, I kept thinking about you."

I took a deep breath. "So, do you think we should lose
sleep tonight alone, or together?"

We both laughed, but neither of us answered the question. Later on that day we decided to spend the night together. We agreed that my attendant would sleep in Judy's
bed in the cabin so we could have privacy in the van.

I waited naked under the sleeping bag. I had lit a candle
on the dashboard of the van. My attendant waited with me
until Judy came.

The door to the van opened gently. "Knock, knock." Judy

pushed a small cooler in ahead of her. "I brought my food with me in case I need a refueling snack, okay? I have to eat a lot of protein."

"That's great! Nothing like being prepared." I nodded to my attendant that she could leave.

Judy undressed and climbed into bed with me. We talked and giggled nervously for a while. She told me she taught English to Chinese immigrants, and that she was getting her Master's in teaching English as a second language. I told her I was writing a book, and I told her all about the farm. She told me she was interested in linguistics. I told her I was terrible in languages but I was very interested in her.

Then it got quiet, and we looked into each other's eyes for a long time. We kissed, first tentatively, then deeply. The sleeping bag became much too hot although it was below fifty degrees outside in the September mountain weather. She stroked my body and helped me move my hands to touch her. I blew her soft kisses. We made love, laughed, and talked until it began to grow light outside, and fell asleep in each other's arms.

When I returned home at the end of the festival, I realized that to my delight, Judy had left her sleeping bag in my van. I knew that would mean I would have to call her in Boston that evening. I smiled thinking about calling Judy as I unpacked and began to open the pile of mail that had come while I was gone. To my surprise, in the mail there was a job announcement from the Boston Self Help Center looking for a director. There were also two messages on my answering machine from two different friends telling me about the same job, and encouraging me to apply for it because they "really needed someone like you." I rubbed my crystal hard, with the help of my cat, Dianna, who also seemed to like to rub my crystal. I rewrote my resume and mailed it.

Several days later I received a thick envelope from Judy in

the mail. It contained a street map of Boston. She wanted me to know where she lived, and she wanted me to come visit. Neither of us liked long distance relationships, but I felt that since I owned the farm, perhaps she might want to move to New York. I insisted that she come visit me first.

Two days before she came, two women who had committed to moving to the farm called and said they had changed their minds. Without other women sharing living expenses, I would be unable to continue meeting my mortgage payments. The women executors of Barbara Deming's estate who were holding the mortgage had already threatened to foreclose if I fell any further behind than I already was.

When Judy came to visit, I realized that no matter how good our relationship might become, there would be too many economic and physical stresses to overcome if we stayed at Beechtree. I asked my dearest friends what they thought of my moving to Boston. They all said that they'd miss me but that things seemed too hard there for me now, and maybe it was time for me to leave.

I began researching attendant care in Boston. I found out that I could be part of a personal care assistance program through the local Independent Living Center, which would allow me to hire, train and pay attendants of my choice. I visited Judy several times, and found a roommate and an apartment. I hated losing the farm, but I knew I was gaining work possibilities and a wonderful lover.

All of the apartments were inaccessible, so I decided to begin making Boston accessible by building a ramp. I borrowed money for the lumber, and took a bunch of my friends with me to help me move in and build the ramp. Judy gave my cousin, Carol, an architect, the measurements of the steps over the phone, and Carol drew up blueprints for a thirty-foot ramp and mailed them to me.

We arrived in Boston with a load of wood and a van load of furniture. My friends carried me in and began building. We called many of Judy's friends, and women's shelters and bookstores asking for volunteers to help with the construction. I was unable to leave the house until the ramp was completed. Every day it rained, and every day a crew of women sawed wood and pounded nails in the rain. Eight days later, the last nail was pounded in, just in time for me to go to a Holly Near concert.

The Boston Self Help Center interviewed me three times and offered me the position of director. The Center provided peer counseling, information, referrals and advocacy services for persons with disabilities and their families, employers, co-workers and friends. The Center also did sensitivity training and education in the areas of disability and chronic illness. They were offering me a position which would *pay* me to do much of the political and social change work that I had been doing most of my life merely in order to survive. I was thrilled. It had been so long since I was allowed to work. I felt a rush of grief over all the years of feeling stripped of the dignity of working. I was afraid to take the chance of accepting the job, because it could all be taken away again, but my excitement won out and I accepted.

Massachusetts had several different programs to provide attendant care to people with disabilities who were working. I was able to maintain my attendant care, my disability and medical benefits, and still work. Some of the pieces of legislation that I had worked on over ten years earlier had finally been written into law. There was a law allowing a trial work period for persons on Social Security, to encourage people to attempt to work and maintain their benefits until they proved they were able to continue to function in a job.

Several of the clients at the Boston Self Help Center needed therapy in addition to the peer counseling we provided. I began to see a few of them privately to provide those services. In addition, several of my attendants made referrals to me. Within a year I had a part-time art therapy practice. Nearly all of my clients were women. A few of them had disabilities. Most of my clients were women with past abuse histories. Some of them were able to pay, and others did work exchange. Those clients referred other clients, and eventually I ran several groups. I was fulfilling my dream to be an art therapist.

Periodically I would think of Dawn, the girl I had helped care for in Los Angeles, and miss her terribly. I often did telephone searches to try to locate her or members of her family by calling information in various major cities across the country. I knew that at age seven she had been diagnosed with neurofibromatosis. As a result she was deaf in one ear and had back and joint problems. Another symptom of the disease was that her skin developed large patchy discolorations. One day when Dawn was about fifteen I had gotten lucky and located her mother. Dawn and I had some brief, polite conversations that seemed a bit strange. When she was sixteen, I got a frantic phone call from her. She said she needed to come visit me. I knew that she had been having a difficult time since she was thirteen; we had talked about a little of it on the phone. In fact, she had left home for a while.

I didn't know why she wanted to come see me, but I didn't care, and was overjoyed at the prospect of seeing her again. I was glad I had decided not to have a child of my own. There was no need to. Dawn was as close to me as I could ever want any child to be. When I couldn't find her for five years, I had felt like I had lost my daughter.

I waited with anticipation as streams of people filed off the plane. This small bleached blonde in high heels, mountains of makeup and a white fox fur coat bent over and hugged and kissed me, squealing "Hi!" I choked from the perfume. We drove from the airport with Dawn talking nonstop about her parents and her sister and where she lived in Oregon.

When we got home, Dawn changed into a long negligee and fancy robe. We ate lasagna while she asked me thousands of questions about my life. She had no problems with my being a lesbian now. In fact, she had been lovers with a few women several years earlier. She seemed to adjust quickly to the changes there had been in my disability. It was fun, but there was a tension in the air.

After dinner we went to unpack her clothes. She told me more about what her life had been like out on the streets. She had left home when she was thirteen because she wasn't getting along with her mother, and didn't feel that there was enough room for her in the trailer they lived in. She had gotten into drugs, and finally prostitution for nearly two years. Then she had gone home when she was fifteen to live with her sister and had started therapy because sometimes she just felt mean and angry and didn't know why, and other times she would get very scared. She said she had started remembering how different boyfriends of her mother's had made her have sex with them when she was little. Just when Dawn had started to do better, her sister and her sister's boyfriend broke up. Her sister had to move out, and couldn't take Dawn with her. So she had found herself out on her own again at age fifteen. She was able to find a little work, but needed the help of several male friends. They took care of her and gave her presents in exchange for "favors." She showed me the outfits she wore for them and some of the things they bought her.

She talked on and on long into the night, and I listened with all my heart and soul, trying to stay present for her and not give in to my own rage at all those men who had hurt her so much. I felt guilty as if I had abandoned her, yet I knew I had had no choice. I remembered reading about several women with disabilities losing their children to foster care or adoption because Medicaid wouldn't pay for per-

sonal assistance to help them take care of their children. If I
had taken Dawn with me from California, Social Services
could have done the same to me and taken her away. After
all, she wasn't legally my child, and even if she had been,
they wouldn't have provided me with attendant services to
help me care for her. But, I knew that I would have been a
better mother for Dawn than her own mother. I knew her
mother loved her, but her mother couldn't give the emotional stability that Dawn needed in her life. I knew I could
have provided that much for Dawn, and more, since I too
had a disability.

The next day I took her to a Take Back the Night March
that was blessedly happening in Boston at just the right
time. As Dawn listened to the rally, I could see her getting
angry. She heard women speaking out about sex abuse, and
prostitutes speaking out proudly about how they had survived the streets. She heard women shouting that "Yes
means yes, and no means no." She heard about not having to
paint yourself up for men, and about being able to be safe on
the streets.

As the women began to march, Dawn kicked off her heels
and took off her fur coat, plopping them in my lap saying,
"Hold these. I've got to go march with these women."
Friends I ran into at the march looked surprised at the sight
of me with a fox fur lap robe, but I didn't care.

Over the next several weeks, I held Dawn sobbing in my
lap, reliving the memories of her early abuse and prostitution. I fought with her for her own identity. I took her to
Forty-second Street in New York City because she wanted
to see what the "big-time" street life looked like. She would
wear black leather and chains one day, and pleated woolen
skirts the next. She worked at a local drugstore for some
cash while she was with me, and solicited several sexual of-
fers from local businessmen, but later turned them down.
Dawn got calls from the men in Oregon that had "kept" her.
She also got a few calls from a nineteen year old named

Greg who was in the Navy. She said he didn't "keep her" like the other men did, but he was real nice. She curled my hair and we ate junk food and watched movies on TV together. She got mad at me for being old; she got mad at me for not understanding, and sometimes she got mad at me for understanding. I was getting pelted with many years of anger in a short amount of time. I learned to struggle with her to make up for the years of parenting I hadn't had the chance to do. Some of her struggle reminded me of some of my own struggles. I had also gone through sexual identity confusion after the man had molested me in the van. In a world of disability oppression and stereotypes, I struggled daily for my own voice. Perhaps now I could help my surrogate child struggle for hers.

We came back to Boston and went shopping for reasonable clothes Dawn could afford, and then we went to Saks, Bloomingdale's, and other stores she could never afford without the help of her men friends. Dawn liked to try on the most expensive dress in every store. She tried on a white gown in Saks that she loved. I went back to the store without her to buy it, and gave it to her as a present just before she got on the plane to leave Boston.

She burst into tears as she opened the box. "Oh! I could get married in this dress! I could get married in this dress, couldn't I?"

"Yes, you could." We hugged and kissed goodbye.

Months later I got a phone call from Dawn. "Hello, Connie? This is Mrs. Dawn Robinson! You know that dress you bought me? Well, I got married in it! I married Greg. He's really nice, and I checked out his whole family and nobody's ever been divorced. They're real faithful. And now that I'm a Navy wife, they pay all my medical expenses, even therapy."

"Well, isn't that wonderful!" I smiled through my tears.

After I hung up the phone, I thought about my own old

buried desires to want to be married. I had always wanted to marry Ron, even if he didn't want to be monogamous. When he had proposed marriage the first time, I had accepted, but he hadn't been serious. Years later when he proposed several times, I refused because I didn't think he was capable of that kind of commitment. I think I also refused because I didn't want to be "owned" the way one is when they're married. When I had become a lesbian, I had been relieved that no one in the community got married. When it then became the trend for lesbians to make commitments and have marriage ceremonies, I cringed. I supposed being lovers with Judy was the most like a marriage that I could ever imagine, in the positive ways, and the least like marriage in the negative ways. We were completely there for each other financially, spiritually, emotionally and physically, but did not own each other. We made mutual decisions with one another based on what was better for each individual. We at least strived to support one another even when we personally disagreed with the other's choice. At the same time, we were honest with each other about our opinions. Even though I never got married, Glenn had been wrong when he had said that no one could ever marry me. He could not bear the thought of becoming partnered with me because of my disability, yet I have had many committed lovers who have come close to that partnership. Of all of them, Judy had come the closest. My thoughts turned back to Dawn. Having her back in my life provided a richness and a completeness. I wondered if she would ever have children, and if so what it would be like to be a surrogate grandmother.

Boston proved to be an interesting city. While it was smaller and more manageable then New York, the population seemed more transient. I had better access to health food stores, and I finally got an adapted computer. Through Children's Hospital I got a sophisticated electric wheelchair from Sweden, called a Permobil, which enabled me to reposition myself. This was a Goddess-send because my disability was causing more and more pain as it progressed. I needed to reposition myself every ten to fifteen minutes in order to avoid cramping and pressure sores. The chair allowed me to drive with my thumb, move my legs or my back, or tilt the chair, or raise it up in the air, all with a puff-and-sip tube in my mouth. I could steer with the puff-and-sip, and change speeds also.

My mother and I had grown closer over the years. I came to better understand what she had gone through as a young women confronted with a child with a severe disability. It would have been very different for her and for me if personal assistance had been available at that time for children. One day she flew to Boston to spend a day with me. I met her at the airport at eight o'clock in the morning. We had a quick breakfast at a croissant shop at the airport, then left to shop at Copley Place. We shopped for hours, and then I took her to lunch.

"So, how do you like Boston, Mom?"

"It's nice! It's not as hectic as New York."

"I tried that recipe that you gave me for the quick sauce. Judy loved it."

"Yeah, it's easy. You can put any vegetables in it. Cauliflower, eggplant, fried squash. Your father loves it!"

"It's an easy thing to make when you're really busy. You were busy a lot when we were growing up."

"Yeah, I had a lot to do with you and your sister, and your brother was very active, and your father needed a lot of help with his work."

"I don't know how you did it," I said, looking at her intently.

"I don't either. I thought I would lose my mind sometimes, everybody saying, 'Ma, Ma, Ma! I need this. I need that.'"

"I'm sorry it was so hard, Mom."

"Me too. I think it was hard on all of us. I'm only glad that you're doing well. I think it's great."

"There should have been personal assistant services for children like us so you could've had a break. I'm working on getting a federal bill passed that will provide funding for personal assistant services for anyone with a disability, no matter what age."

Mom nodded.

We then toured Fanueil Hall and drove around the river. We came back to the house to rest, and then we went out to dinner. She went back to the airport laden with bags of souvenirs and clothes and a big smile on her face. She kissed me goodbye and I said, "I love you, Mom."

"I love you too, Conn. The house looks beautiful. You're doing great."

I took advantage of the fact that Boston has one of the world's largest concentrations of medical centers and found a neurologist at Tuft's New England Medical Center who knew a lot about my disability. He told me that they had recently changed the name from Werdnig-Hoffman's Disease, Type II, to Spinal Muscular Atrophy, Type III. I resented it. Nobody had asked me if they could change my name. I mean if you're Italian they wouldn't all of a sudden say, now we're calling you a Martian or a Dandelion. It still meant the same thing, that the anterior horn cells of my spine did not send the nerve messages across to my voluntary muscles. The neurologist wanted to perform surgery on me to straighten my spine so that there would be more room for my lungs and internal organs. I felt threatened because I knew that I would not survive that kind of surgery. I was suffering from stomach ulcers, asthma, digestive difficulties and poor circulation. To have my spine fused would mean having to stay lying down on a bed for three months. The chances of contracting pneumonia were very high. And the chances of my respiratory muscles permanently atrophying, leading to permanent ventilator dependency were even higher. I asked him what the chances of survival would be. He said that unless my spine was straightened I would die anyway. I told him, "Two of my friends with Werdnig-Hoffman's died from that surgery. Another of my friends with Werdnig-Hoffman's, which you now call Spinal Muscular Atrophy, had that surgery, and her spine curved anyway. But, now that she has metal in her spine, she's in great pain all the time. She's on several prescription pain medications around the clock. I am going to be forty years old this year. Aren't you interested in how I've survived this long? Don't you want to know what's keeping me alive and active?"

"You need to have this surgery. There's nothing I can do for you if you don't have it. I'm going to call and make the appointment with the orthopedist." He picked up the phone, dialed and started talking to someone.

When he hung up I told him, "I'm not going to go to an orthopedist. I see a chiropractor. I have for years. It helps a good deal with my neck vertebra, which move out of place often because of the weak neck muscles that go along with this disability. When I see the chiropractor regularly, I have no headaches."

"Well, witchcraft helps too, I suppose . . ." He finished writing out the referral slip for the orthopedist. "By the way, I'd like you to get some blood drawn today and schedule an electromyogram—."

Judy interrupted him asking, "Will that be for information to help Connie or for your own research?"

"Research! Who said anything about research?"

Judy pressed, "How will an electromyogram help Connie?"

The doctor turned to me and said, "We would like to have you take part in one of our studies. You have a sister with SMA, don't you?"

I nodded.

"Well, we want your sister to contribute blood also. We

can arrange to get her blood from New York. We're trying to isolate the gene which causes this disability. You know, you people are quite smart." He turned to Judy, my lover and said, "Do you know that people with Spinal Muscular Atrophy are often close to genius?"

"Why do you want to isolate the gene?" I asked.

"Well, so that we can screen out for the gene. Wouldn't it be wonderful if a woman could have amniocentesis and avoid having a child with Spinal Muscular Atrophy?"

"No! I don't think it would be wonderful at all. I'm glad I was born." I dropped the referral slip on the floor and said goodbye. Judy followed me down the hall. When we got into the elevator, I broke into sobs. This man was one of the top researchers in the world for my disability, and all he wanted to do was annihilate my kind from the face of the earth. I thought about being close to genius. I thought about the adults I worked with in Liberty, New York at the Bennett Residence. Some of them had IQs of three, yet they were beautiful and funny and creative. It didn't matter whether I was a genius or not, I was living and breathing, and I had a right to survive. Even if I couldn't breathe on my own, I had a right to survive! After all, Curtis Brewer, my lawyer, lived on a respirator. "When will they learn, Judy?" I sobbed. "When will they learn that eliminating life isn't the same as eliminating disability?"

A few months later, I was invited to speak at the National Lesbian and Gay Pride March on Washington. Judy went with me and my attendant. The trip was a struggle since the airline dropped my wheelchair twice, smashing all the battery connections. A flight engineer rewired the chair when they dropped it in New York, and gave Judy extra parts. Judy rewired it after they dropped it again in Washington.

As I faced the murmuring crowd of three hundred thousand people gathered at the morning rally, I thought of how far we had come, and how much farther we had to go. There was a ramp for me to get up onto the stage, but it was in the back of the stage, and poorly designed, it was so steep that it took four people to help me up.

"Hi! It's good to be here. How about you, are you glad to be here?" A shout came up from the crowd. Their energy was enormous and took me by surprise. "I'm proud to be here. Proud that I'm a lesbian, proud that I'm disabled, and proud to like my body. I want to talk to you about ableism. Do you know what ableism is? Ableism is the disease that causes us to hate what's 'different.' It's what homophobia and sexism and racism are about. Ableism says that those who are more 'able' should have more rights, more power, and more money than those who are less able." The crowd became silent. "We have all grown up in this country with this view. Ableism supports the patriarchal system which says that AIDS research must take second priority to national defense, just like all other disease research. This country hates people with any illness or disabling conditions, not just people with AIDS. We need to turn that around. We need cures and preventions for people with AIDS and all people with illnesses and disabilities. We need money for attendant care, equipment and housing for all people who need them. There's plenty of money out there." People shouted, "Yeah! Yeah!"

"We need to stop committing ableism amongst ourselves. Each time you look in the mirror and say to yourself, 'I'm too fat,' or 'my skin is ugly,' or, 'I'm too skinny,' you are committing ableism. Be proud of your difference. What would a forest be like if every single tree and every leaf were identical? I have seen some very beautiful trees with twisted or broken branches.

"I'm tired of being ashamed. I'm proud of being a lesbian! And I'm proud of being disabled. It's *'nice'* that they built a ramp so I could get up here to speak to you, but why are the steps in the front and the ramp in the back? Next time I want to see that ramp out front! I love you all, and I want you to love yourselves and each other."

I felt lifted up into the air by the cheering. I did not feel like a performer, or an act in a sideshow. I felt like a treasured member of a great throng, and we all agreed.

Selected Titles from Seal Press

PAST DUE: *A Story of Disability, Pregnancy and Birth* by Anne Finger. 0-931188-87-3, $10.95. In this eloquent and deeply moving book, a writer disabled by polio explores the complexities of disability and reproductive rights through a riveting account of her pregnancy and childbirth experience.

THE BLACK WOMEN'S HEALTH BOOK: *Speaking for Ourselves*, Expanded Second Edition, edited by Evelyn C. White. 1-878067-40-0, $16.95. In this pioneering anthology, black women writers and health care providers address today's health issues and testify to the determination of black women to get well and stay well. Contributors include Faye Wattleton, Byllye Y. Avery, Alice Walker, Angela Y. Davis, Toni Morrison, bell hooks and many more.

YOU DON'T HAVE TO TAKE IT!: *A Woman's Guide to Confronting Emotional Abuse at Work* by Ginny NiCarthy, Naomi Gottlieb and Sandra Coffman. 1-878067-35-4, $14.95. This groundbreaking book provides practical advice and exercises to help women recognize abusive situations and respond with constructive action, including confrontation and workplace organizing.

SHE WHO WAS LOST IS REMEMBERED: *Healing From Incest Through Creativity* edited by Louise M. Wisechild. 1-878067-09-5, $18.95. This collection presents the work of more than thirty women visual artists, musicians, and writers, along with essays by each contributor on how she used creativity to mend from childhood abuse.

LESBIAN COUPLES: *Creating Healthy Relationships for the 90s* by D. Merilee Clunis and G. Dorsey Green. 1-878067-37-0, $12.95. A new edition of the highly acclaimed and popular guide for lesbian couples. Topics include living arrangements, coming out to family and friends, resolving conflict and understanding each other—accompanied by real life examples and helpful problem-solving techniques.

THE MOTHER I CARRY: *A Memoir of Healing from Emotional Abuse* by Louise M. Wisechild. 1-878067-38-9, $12.95. This stunningly honest and beautifully written autobiography explores the author's relationship with her emotionally abusive mother.

SEAL PRESS, founded in 1976 to provide a forum for women writers and feminist issues, has many other titles in stock: fiction, self-help books, anthologies, international literature and mysteries. You may order directly from us at 3131 Western Avenue, Suite 410, Seattle, Washington 98121 (add 15% of total book order for shipping and handling). Write to us for a free catalog.